D0421931

FIND YOUR WAY TO INNER PEACE...

Our turmoil-ridden world has made many people unsatisfied with themselves. The author of this enlightening book has written on the various ways that Yoga philosophy can lead you to a deeper, happier life. A true Spiritual Master, he answers questions like: What is Yoga? Who is fit for Yoga? What is the aim of life?

The Voice of Silence

The Voice of Silence need not and will not give us the same thing always.

As we evolve, it gives us better, higher and more fulfilling light.

YOGA AND THE SPIRITUAL LIFE:
THE JOURNEY OF INDIA'S SOUL

SRI CHINMOY

Time

O Time, you go your own way.
My God shall remain my eternal now.

YOGA

AND THE

SPIRITUAL LIFE

THE JOURNEY OF
INDIA'S SOUL

SRI CHINMOY

YOGA AND THE SPIRITUAL LIFE:
THE JOURNEY OF INDIA'S SOUL

by
SRI CHINMOY

Copyright © 1974 by Sri Chinmoy

ISBN 0-88497-040-X
Library of Congress
Catalogue No. 74-81309

Published and Printed by:
Agni Press
84-47 Parsons Boulevard
Jamaica, New York

PART ONE:
SPIRITUAL AND PHILOSOPHICAL
ARTICLES

PART TWO:
QUESTIONS AND ANSWERS

PART THREE:
RELIGION (MAINLY HINDUISM)

****

If you do not know the capacity of your mind, you have not missed much.

If you do not know the capacity of your heart, you have missed much.

If you do not know the capacity of your soul, you have missed all.

PREFACE

In this book, the illumined spiritual Master Sri Chinmoy presents a fresh and original perspective on various aspects of Yoga and the spiritual life. Written in a practical vein, it offers the newcomer as well as the advanced seeker some deep, penetrating insights into Eastern mysticism and philosophy.

The latter half of the book contains questions and answers on the soul and the inner life. These have been drawn from the thousands of questions Sri Chinmoy has been asked over the years during his university lectures and public meditations.

Love

*Pure Love and untold misery do not and
   cannot live together.*
*Pure love is the body's constant oneness
   with the soul's flood of delight.*

PART ONE:

SPIRITUAL AND PHILOSOPHICAL ARTICLES

Mind and Heart

The mind of reason fails.
The heart of faith sails.
The mind of reason is man's mortality.
The heart of faith is God's Immortality.

MAN AND GOD

Man and God are eternally one. Like God, man is infinite; like man, God is finite. There is no yawning gulf between man and God. Man is the God of tomorrow; God, the man of yesterday and today.

As God is in Heaven, even so is He on earth. He is here, there and everywhere. Each human being has a God of his own. There is no human being without a God. The total atheist does not believe in God. But fortunately he believes, or rather unfortunately he *has* to believe, in a certain idea, some concept of order or disorder. And that very idea, that concept, is nothing but God.

Freedom, absolute freedom, must be given each individual soul to discover its own path. Mistakes along the path of spirituality are not at all deplorable, for mistakes are simply lesser truths. We are not proceeding from falsehood to truth. We are proceeding from the least revealed truth to the most revealed truth.

Until we have realised God and have become one with God, we have to call upon Him as Master, Guide, Friend and so on. According to our relationship with Him, our attitude toward Him may vary. This is of no consequence. What is of supreme importance is that we love God as our very own. In our sincere love of God, we shall be inspired spontaneously to worship Him.

Here we shall have to know which kind of worship is for us, which kind is in harmony with the development and inclination of our soul. The realisation of absolute oneness with God is the highest form of worship. Next in the descending line is meditation. Lower is the seat for prayers and invocations. The lowest form of worship is the worship of God in things mundane.

When I think that the flute and the Flutist are two different things, I think of myself as God's servant and Him as my Master. When I feel that the flute has a part of its Master's consciousness, I feel that I am God's child and He is my Father. Finally, when I realise that the flute and the Flutist are but one, the Flutist appears as the Spirit and I as Its creative Force.

Man has to realise God in this body here on earth. India's great poet Kabir said:

> "If your bonds be not broken, whilst living, what hope of deliverance in death?
> "It is an empty dream that the soul shall have union with Him because it has passed from the body;
> "If He is found now, He is found then;

"If not, we do go to dwell in the city of Death."

Sisters and brothers, do not sink into the abyss of despair, even if you have, at the moment, no clear aspiration for God-realisation. Just start on your journey upward, inward and forward — upward to see God's Dream, inward to possess God's Dream, forward to become God's Dream. This Dream is the Dream of absolute Fulfilment.

Countless are those who launch onto the path of the inner life only after receiving innumerable blows or after wandering far and wide in the deserts of life. So he is indeed happy and blessed who places his body, mind, heart and soul — like flowers — at the Feet of the Lord before the advent of blows. It is true that the teeming clouds of worldliness cover up our yet unlit mind. It is equally true that the volcano of the seeker's concentration and the hydrogen bomb of his meditation can and will destroy the clouds, the age-long mists of Ignorance.

May I say a word to those who are married and have great family responsibilities? To your utter amazement, all such responsibilities will be transformed into golden opportunities the moment you try to see God in your children, the moment you realise that you are serving God in your self-sacrifice. In its ability to fulfil the husband, to establish him divinely in the boundless expanse of matter, to raise his consciousness into the realm of Spirit, the untiring and spontaneous sacrifice of the wife has no substitute. In its ability to inundate the wife's soul with the Peace of the Beyond, to beckon her heart to the ever-blazing Sun of Infinity, to transmute her life into Immortality's Song, the husband's promise has no substitute. And those who are single can rest assured that they are singled out to run the fastest along the spiritual path. Inseparable are their aspiration and God's Inspiration.

When we try to see deep within, when we try to live an inner life, we may encounter difficulties all around. We cry out, "Look, God, now that we have turned toward You, we have to take so many tests!" Finding no way out, we are perturbed. But why should we be? It cannot escape our remembrance that we have endured misfortunes in our life. Before we entered the spiritual life, despondency proved to be our constant companion. Now we are at least in a better position since we have the capacity to recognize the ferocious tiger of worldliness. Let us take restlessness and weakness as tests.

Why should God test us? He does anything but that. He, being the Merciful, warns us of the imminent danger. But if we take these warnings as tests, then to pass the test, we have to pray to God. Merely by thinking of the difficulties and dangers we can never pass the examination. To pass a test in school, we have to study hard. Similarly, to pass an inner examination, we have to cultivate more sincerity and feed the flame of aspiration.

4

During meditation we have to be very careful. At times the mind wants to indulge in certain worldly and emotional ideas and thoughts, but we must not permit the mind to do so. During meditation everything is intense and, if we indulge in evil thoughts, the effects become more serious and more dangerous than otherwise. We grow weaker the moment the mind becomes prey to self-indulgent thoughts. It is the very nature of our lower mind to deceive us. But our tears and our heart's mounting flame will always come to our rescue.

Man and God are one. All men belong to the same family. We are all one. A genuine seeker must not listen to the absurd arguments of sceptics. They do not have even a pennyworth of spiritual knowledge. They are unaware of the fact that they are unconsciously making a parade of their naked stupidity. They say, "If we are all one, then how is it that when you have a headache, I do not? When my hunger is appeased, how is it that yours is not?" In reply, let us ask them how it is that when they have a leg wound, their head does not hurt as well, since both are part of the same body. The universal consciousness is within us all. If we are not conscious of it, that does not mean that it does not exist. My body is my own. But do I feel pain in my leg when my head suffers from a headache? No. But if I am aware of the Divine Consciousness which pervades my whole body, undoubtedly I shall feel the same pain all over my body. Here the individual soul is my head and the collective soul is my whole body. To feel the entire world as our very own we have first to feel God as our very own.

> Man is Infinity's Heart.
> Man is Eternity's Breath.
> Man is Immortality's Life.

WITHIN US IS OUR GOAL

We are God's all-fulfilling Dream. Our within is God's boundless Plenitude. Our goal is Infinity's Heart and Immortality's Breath. Our goal is within our very body.

In the physical world the mother tells the child who his father is. In the spiritual world our aspiration tells us who our God is. Who is God? God is an infinite Consciousness. He is also the self-illumining Light. There is no human being who does not own within himself this infinite Consciousness and this self-illumining Light.

If we want to see anything in the outer world, in addition to keeping our eyes wide open, we need light — either sunlight or electric light or some other kind of light. But in the inner world we need no light whatsoever. Even with our eyes closed we can see God, the self-illumining Light.

God is not something to be obtained from outside. God is that very thing which can be unfolded from within.

In the ordinary life each human being has millions and millions of questions to ask. In his spiritual life, a day dawns when he feels that there is only one question worth asking: "Who am I?" The answer of answers is: "I am not the body, but I am the Inner Pilot."

How is it that a man does not know himself, something which ought to be the easiest of all his endeavours? He does not know himself precisely because he identifies himself with the ego and not with his real Self. What compels him to identify himself with this pseudo-self? It is ignorance. And what tells him that the real Self is not and can never be the ego? It is his Self-search. What he sees in the inmost recesses of his heart is his real Self, his God. Eventually this seeing must transform itself into becoming.

The other day one of my students said to me, "I can't think of God. My mind becomes restless."

"What do you do then?" I asked.

"Why, I just think of the world."

"Now tell me, when you think of the world with all its activities, can you even for a second think of God?"

"No, never."

"So, my young friend, is it not absurd that when you think of God, restlessness takes your mind away from God, but when you drink deep the pleasures of the world, restlessness does not take your mind away and place it at the Feet of the Lord? No, this should never be. If you have genuine hunger for spiritual food, the same restlessness, or what you may call 'uneasiness,' will take your mind speedily and dynamically and place it in your heart where it can drink the Nectar of divine Peace and Satisfaction.

"To be sure, your mind cannot do two things at a time. If you are thinking of God with an implicit faith, if the flame of aspiration is burning within your heart, your outer restlessness-monkey, however mischievous it may be, will not dare to touch you, much less pinch or bite you. You cannot look with full attention at both your shoulders at the same time. Similarly, when you clearly see your God within, you cannot see the ignorance-tiger of the outer world."

What we have to do first is to see the ego, then touch and catch the ego and finally transform the ego. In the spiritual life, when the ego enters into us and bothers us, we have to think of ourselves as the Brahman, the One without a second, and we have to feel ourselves as the all-pervading Consciousness. Then the ego disappears into nothingness.

We all know that the mind plays an important role in our outer life as well as in our spiritual life. Therefore, we must not discard the mind. Rather, what we should do is be always conscious of the mind. The mind becomes restless, but that does not mean that we have to punish it all the time. If the master of the house comes to learn that his old servant has recently formed the habit of stealing, he does not immediately dismiss the servant. The servant's past sincerity and dedication are still fresh in his mind. He waits and observes unnoticed and unconcerned, feeling that his servant will turn over a new leaf. In the meantime, the servant becomes aware that his master has come to know of his misconduct, and he stops stealing. He goes one step further: to please his master, he works even more sincerely and devotedly than he did before. Similarly, when we become aware of the mind's restless activities and tricks, we have to be silent for some time and observe the mind quite unconcerned. Before long, we shall see that our mind, the thief, will feel ashamed of its conduct. We must not forget that during that time we have to think of ourselves as the soul and not as the body, for the soul alone can be master of the mind. The soul alone is our true identity. At the appointed hour, the mind will start to listen to the dictates of the soul.

Action and inaction. According to the *Gita,* we have to see action in inaction, and inaction in action. What does this mean? It means that, while acting, we have to feel within ourselves a sea of peace and serenity. While we are without activity, we have to feel within us a dynamo of creative energy. Let us not think of actions as our own. If we can do this, our actions will be more real and more effective. When a servant cooks for his master he does it to the best of his capacity. Why? To get his master's appreciation and favour. In the same way, if we act to please our soul, the Inner Pilot, we shall be able to act most devotedly and most successfully.

Our Goal is within us. To reach that Goal we have to take to the spiritual life. In the spiritual life, the thing that is most needed is awareness or consciousness. Without this, everything is a barren desert. When we enter into a dark place, we take a flashlight or some other light in order to know where we are going. If we want to know about our unlit life, we have to take the help of our consciousness. Let us go deeper into the matter. We know that the sun illumines the world. But how are we aware of it? We are aware of it through our consciousness, which is self-revealing. The functioning of the sun is not self-revealing. It is our consciousness of the sun that makes us feel that the sun illumines the world. It is our consciousness that is self-revealing in everything. And this consciousness is an infinite Sea of Delight. When we drink even a drop of water from the earthly sea, it tastes salty. In the same way, during our meditation, if we can drink even a tiny drop from the Sea of Delight, we shall definitely taste Delight. This Delight is Nectar. Nectar is Immortality.

Compassion and Surrender

We shall never find any replacement
*   for God's Compassion.*
We shall never find anything to equal
*   our conscious surrender to God's*
*   loving Care.*

OUR PEACE IS WITHIN

No price is too great to pay for inner peace. Peace is the harmonious control of life. It is vibrant with life-energy. It is a power that easily transcends all our worldly knowledge. Yet it is not separate from our earthly existence. If we open the right avenues within, this peace can be felt here and now.

Peace is eternal. It is never too late to have peace. Time is always ripe for that. We can make our life truly fruitful if we are not cut off from our Source, which is the Peace of Eternity.

The greatest misfortune that can come to a human being is to lose his inner peace. No outer force can rob him of it. It is his own thoughts, his own actions, that rob him of it.

Our greatest protection lies not in our material achievements and resources. All the treasure of the world is emptiness to our divine soul. Our greatest protection lies in our soul's communion with the all-nourishing and all-fulfilling Peace. Our soul lives in Peace and lives for Peace. If we live a life of peace, we are ever enriched and never impoverished. Unhorizoned is our inner peace; like the boundless sky, it encompasses all.

Long have we struggled, much have we suffered, far have we travelled. But the face of peace is still hidden from us. We can discover it if ever the train of our desires loses itself in the Will of the Lord Supreme.

Peace is life. Peace is Bliss eternal. Worries — mental, vital and physical — do exist. But it is up to us whether to accept them or reject them. To be sure, they are not inevitable facts of life. Since our Almighty Father is All-Peace, our common heritage is Peace. It is a Himalayan blunder to widen the broad way of future repentance by misusing and neglecting the golden opportunities that are presented to us. We must resolve here and now, amidst all our daily activities, to throw ourselves, heart and soul, into the Sea of Peace. He is mistaken who thinks that peace will, on its own, enter into him near the end of his life's journey. To hope to achieve peace without spirituality or meditation is to expect water in the desert.

For peace of mind, prayer is essential. To pray to God for peace with full concentration and singleness of devotion even for five minutes is more important than to spend long hours in carefree and easy-going meditation. Now, how to pray? With tears in our hearts. Where to pray? In a lonely place. When to pray? The moment our inner being wants us to pray. Why to pray? This is the question of questions. We have to pray if we want our aspirations to be fulfilled by God. What can we expect from God beyond this? We can expect Him to make us understand everything: everything in nothing and nothing in everything, the Full in the Void and the Void in the Full.

We must always discriminate. We have to feel that the outer world which attracts our attention is ephemeral. To have something everlasting, to attain to a rocklike foundation in life, we have to turn toward God. There is no alternative. And there is no better moment to take that turn than when we feel most helpless.

> To feel oneself helpless is good.
> Better to cultivate the spirit of self-surrender.
> Best to be the conscious instrument of God.

Everything depends on the mind, consciously or unconsciously, including the search for peace. The function of the mind is to remove the cloud of doubt. The function of purity in the mind is to destroy the teeming clouds of worldliness and the ties of ignorance. If there is no purity of the mind, there can be no sustained success in the spiritual life.

We own peace only after we have totally stopped finding fault with others. We have to feel the whole world as our very own. When we observe others' mistakes, we enter into their imperfections. This does not help us in the least. Strangely enough, the deeper we plunge, the clearer it becomes to us that the imperfections of others are our own imperfections, but in dif-

15

ferent bodies and minds. Whereas if we think of God, His Compassion and His Divinity enlarge our inner vision of Truth. We must come in the fulness of our spiritual realisation to accept humanity as one family.

We must not allow our past to torment and destroy the peace of our heart. Our present good and divine actions can easily counteract our bad and undivine actions of the past. If sin has the power to make us weep, meditation has undoubtedly the power to give us joy, to endow us with the divine Wisdom.

Our peace is within, and this peace is the basis of our life. So from today let us resolve to fill our minds and hearts with the tears of devotion, the foundation of peace. If our foundation is solid, then no matter how high we raise the superstructure, danger can never threaten us. For peace is below, peace is above, peace is within, peace is without.

WHO IS FIT FOR YOGA?

Who is fit for Yoga? You are fit for Yoga. He is fit for Yoga. I am fit for Yoga. All human beings without exception are fit for Yoga.

The spiritual fitness can be determined by our feeling of oneness, our desire for oneness. The tiniest drop has a right to feel the boundless ocean as its very own, or to cry to have the ocean as its very own. Such is the case with the individual soul and the Universal Soul.

Where is God and where am I? God is on the third floor and I am on the first floor. I come up to the second floor. He comes down to the second floor. We both meet together. I do not forget to wash His Feet with my tears of delight. Nor does He forget to place me in His Heart of infinite Compassion.

What is Yoga? Yoga is self-conquest. Self-conquest is God-realisation. He who practises Yoga does two things with one stroke: he simplifies his whole life and he gets a free access to the Divine.

In the field of Yoga we can never pretend. Our aspiration must ring true. Our whole life must ring true. Nothing is impossible for an ardent aspirant. A higher Power guides his steps. God's adamantine Will is his safest protection. No matter how long or how many times he blunders, he has every right to come back to his own spiritual home. His aspiration is a climbing flame. It has no smoke, it needs no fuel. It is the breath of his inner life. It leads him to the shores of the Golden Beyond. The aspirant, with the wings of his aspiration, soars into the realms of the Transcendental.

God is Infinite and God is Omnipresent. To a genuine aspirant, this is more than mere belief. It is the Reality without a second.

Now let us focus our attention on the spiritual life. It is a mistaken idea that the spiritual life is a life of austerity and a bed of thorns. No, never! We came from the Blissful. To the Blissful we shall return with the spontaneous joy of life. It seems difficult because we cater to our ego. It looks unnatural because we cherish our doubts.

The realisation of God is the goal of our life. It is also our noblest heritage. God is at once our Father and our Mother. As our Father He observes; as our Mother He creates. Like a child, we shall never give up demanding of our Mother, so that we can win our Mother's Love and Grace. How long can a mother go on unheeding her child's cry? Let us not forget that if there is anybody on earth on whom all human beings have a full claim, it is the Mother aspect of the Divine. She is the only strength of our dependence; she is the only strength of our independence. Her Heart, the home of infinitude, is eternally open to each individual.

We should now become acquainted with the eight significant strides that lead a seeker to his destination. These strides are: *Yama,* self-control and moral abstinence; *Niyama,* strict observance of conduct and character; *Asana,* various body postures which help us enter into a higher consciousness; *Pranayama,* systematic breathing to hold a rein on the mind; *Pratyahara,* withdrawal from the sense-life; *Dharana,* the fixation of our consciousness on God, joined by all parts of the body; *Dhyana,* meditation, the untiring express train speeding toward the Goal; and *Samadhi,* trance, the end of Nature's dance, the total merging of our individual consciousness into the infinite Consciousness of the Transcendental Supreme.

Yoga is our union with Truth. There are three unfolding stages of this union. In the first stage man has to feel that God needs him as much as he needs God. In the second stage man has to feel that, without him, God does not exist even for a second. In the third and ultimate stage man has to realise that he and God are not only eternally One, but also equal, all-pervading and all-fulfilling.

Meditation

God has no time to hate the person
 who finds no time to meditate.
But God has all the time to love and
 treasure the person who soulfully
 meditates every day.

THE STRENGTH OF SURRENDER

The present-day world wants individuality. It demands freedom. But true individuality and freedom can breathe only in the Divine. Surrender is the untiring breath of the soul in the Heart of God.

Human individuality shouts in the dark. Earthly freedom cries out in the deserts of life. But absolute surrender universally sings of divine Individuality and Freedom in the Lap of the Supreme.

In surrender we discover the spiritual power through which we can become not only the seers but also the possessors of Truth. This Truth is the omnipotent Power. If we can surrender in absolute silence, we shall ourselves become the Reality of the Real, the Life of the Living, the Centre of true Love, Peace and Bliss. We shall become an incomparable blessing to ourselves.

A lovely child attracts our attention. We love him because he conquers our heart. But do we ask anything from him in return? No! We love him because he is the object of love; he is lovable. In the same way we can and should love

God, for He is the most lovable Being. Spontaneous love for the Divine is surrender, and this surrender is the greatest gift in life. For when we surrender, the Divine in no time gives us infinitely more than we would have asked for.

Surrender is a spiritual miracle. It teaches us how to see God with our eyes closed, how to talk to Him with our mouth shut. Fear enters into our being only when we withdraw our surrender from the Absolute.

Surrender is an unfoldment. It is the unfoldment of our body, mind and heart into the Sun of divine Plenitude within us. Surrender to this inner Sun is the greatest triumph of life. The hound of failure cannot reach us when we are in this Sun. The Prince of Evil fails to touch us when we have realised and founded our oneness with this eternally life-giving Sun.

Surrender and wholeheartedness play together, eat together and sleep together. Theirs is the crown of victory. Calculation and doubt play together, eat together and sleep together. Theirs is the fate that is doomed to disappointment, destined to failure.

India is the land of surrender. This surrender is not a blind submission, but rather the dedication of one's limited self to one's unbounded Self. There are a good many stories in the *Mahabharata* dealing with surrender. They all have great spiritual truth in them. Let me tell you a short but most inspiring and revealing story about Draupadi, who was the Queen of the

Pandavas. While the evil Duhshasana was ruthlessly attempting to disrobe her, she was praying to the Lord to save her. Yet all the while she was holding her garments tightly with her fists. Her surrender was not complete, and her prayer was not granted. Duhshasana continued his efforts to pull off the garments of the unfortunate Queen. But the moment came when Draupadi released her hold on her robes and began to pray to the Lord with hands upraised. "O Lord of my heart, O Boatman of my life, may Thy Will be fulfilled," she prayed. Lo, the strength of her absolute surrender! God's silence broke. His Grace rained down on Draupadi. As Duhshasana tried to pull off her sari, he found that it was endless. His pride had to kiss the dust.

God's all-fulfilling Grace descends only when man's unconditional surrender ascends.

Our surrender is a most precious thing. God alone deserves it. We can offer our surrender to another individual, but only for the sake of realising God. If that individual has reached his Goal, he can help us in our spiritual journey. If, however, we offer ourselves to someone just to satisfy that person, then we are committing a Himalayan blunder. What we should do is offer ourselves unreservedly to the Lord in him.

Every action of ours should be to please God and not to gain applause. Our actions are too secret and sacred to display before others. They are meant for our own progress, achievement and realisation.

There is no limit to our surrender. The more

we surrender, the more we have to surrender. God has given us capacity. According to our capacity He demands manifestation of us. Manifestation beyond our capacity God has never demanded and will never demand.

In man's complete and absolute surrender is his realisation: his realisation of the Self, his realisation of God the Infinite.

MEDITATION:
INDIVIDUAL AND COLLECTIVE

Meditation is the eye that sees the Truth, the heart that feels the Truth and the soul that realises the Truth.

Through meditation the soul becomes fully aware of its evolution in its eternal journey. Through meditation we see the form evolve into the Formless, the finite into the Infinite; and we see the Formless evolve into the form, the Infinite into the finite.

Meditation speaks. It speaks in silence. It reveals. It reveals to the aspirant that matter and spirit are one, quantity and quality are one, the immanent and the transcendent are one. It reveals that life can never be the mere existence of seventy or eighty years between birth and death, but is, rather, Eternity itself. Our birth is a significant incident in God's own existence. And so is our death. In our birth, life lives in the body. In our death, life lives in the spirit.

Meditation: individual and collective. As the individual and the collective are in essence one, even so are meditation individual and collective. We are all children of God. Our body says that we are human. Our soul says that we are divine.

No matter whether we are human or divine, we are one, inevitably and eternally. We are the inseparable parts of the whole. We complete the whole.

Vast is the ocean. You see a part of it. He sees a part of it. I see a part of it. But the full expanse of the ocean is far beyond our gaze. Our vision is limited. But the portion that each of us sees is not and cannot be separated from the entire ocean.

What does an orchestra produce? It produces a symphonic unity. Different notes from different instruments form the symphony. As each instrument plays its own notes, so each individual may meditate in his own way. But ultimately all will arrive at the same goal and the basic realisation of oneness. And this realisation is nothing other than liberation — liberation from bondage, ignorance and death.

Tat twam asi. "That Thou art." This is indeed the secret that can be revealed in meditation. This "Thou" is not the outer man. This "Thou" is our soul, our divinity within. Our unlit and undivine nature tries to make us feel that the body is everything. Our illumined and divine nature makes us feel that our soul, which has no beginning and no ending, is everything. Indeed, it is the soul that is the breath of our existence both in Heaven and on earth.

Self-knowledge and universal Knowledge are not two different things. Everything in the universe becomes ours the moment we realise our Self. And what is this universe? It is the outer expression of our inner achievements. We are our own Saviours. Within us is our salvation. It is we who have to work for our salvation. We are our own fate-makers. To blame others for the unfavourable conditions of our lives is beneath our dignity. Unfortunately, this act of blaming others is one of man's oldest diseases. Adam blamed Eve for his temptation. Poor Eve, what could she do? She also blamed another. No, we must not do that. If action is ours, responsibility is also ours. To try to escape the consequences of our actions is simply absurd. But to be free from committing blunders is wisdom; it is the real illumination. Trials and tribulations are within us and without us. We simply have to ignore them. If this act of ignoring is not effective, we must face them. If that, too, is not enough, we have to conquer them here and now. The paramount problem is how to conquer the trials and tribulations. We can conquer them only by our constant aspiration and meditation. There is no substitute, no alternative.

From meditation, when it is deep and one-pointed, we get spiritual knowledge and pure devotion, which act not only simultaneously but also harmoniously. The path of *Bhakti,* devotion, and the path of *Jnana,* knowledge, lead us ultimately to the same goal. Devotion is not blind faith. It is not an absurd adherence to our inner feeling. It is a matchless process of spiritual unfoldment. Knowledge is not something dry. Neither is it an aggressive power. Knowledge is the food that energizes our earthly and heavenly existence. Devotion is Delight. Knowledge is Peace. Our heart needs Delight and our mind needs Peace, just as God needs us to manifest Himself and we need God to fulfil ourselves.

Meditation: individual and collective. It is easy to meditate individually. The aspirant is fortunate, for no third person stands between him and God's Grace. It is easy to meditate collectively. A student naturally gets joy while he is studying with others in the class. Here also the aspirant is fortunate, for the sincere aspiration of other seekers may inspire him.

True, there are difficulties in meditating individually, for laziness can plague the aspirant. True, there are difficulties in meditating collectively, because there is every possibility that the ignorance and weaknesses of others may unconsciously attack the aspirant's body, mind and heart.

Whether we meditate individually or collectively, there is one thing we absolutely must do: we have to meditate consciously. Making an unconscious effort is like forcing oneself to play football in spite of one's utmost unwillingness. One plays, but gets no joy. Conscious effort is like playing football most willingly. One gets real joy. Similarly, conscious meditation gives us inner Delight from the soul.

Finally, each human being must have the spirit of a divine hero. If he is left alone in the thickest forest, he must have the inner strength to meditate without fear. If he is asked to meditate in Times Square amid crowds of people, he must have the inner strength to meditate without being disturbed in the least. Whether alone or with others, the aspirant must dwell in his meditation unshaken and unafraid.

Gratitude

To receive one thing with joy is to give ten things in return with gratitude.

HAS YOUR SOUL A SPECIAL MISSION?

Your soul has a special mission. Your soul is supremely conscious of it.

Maya, illusion or forgetfulness, makes you feel that you are finite, weak and helpless. This is not true. You are not the body. You are not the senses. You are not the mind. These are all limited. You are the soul, which is unlimited. Your soul is infinitely powerful. Your soul defies all time and space.

Can you ever realise your soul? Can you be fully conscious of your soul and be one with it? Certainly you can. For, in fact, you are nothing other than the soul. It is your soul that represents the natural state of consciousness. But doubt makes it difficult to realise the soul. Doubt is man's fruitless struggle in the outer world. Aspiration is the seeker's fruitful confidence in the inner world. Doubt struggles and struggles. Finally it defeats its own purpose. Aspiration flies upward to the highest. At its journey's end it reaches the Goal. Doubt is based on outer observation. Aspiration is founded on inner experience. Doubt ends in failure because it lives in the finite physical mind. Aspiration ends in success because it lives in the ever-climbing soul. A life of aspiration is a life of Peace. A life of aspiration is a life of Bliss. A life of aspiration is a life of divine Fulfilment.

To know what your special mission is, you have to go deep within. Hope and courage must accompany you on your tireless journey. Hope will awaken your inner divinity. Courage will make your inner divinity flower. Hope will inspire you to dream of the Transcendental. Courage will inspire you to manifest the Transcendental here on earth.

To feel what your special mission is, you have always to create. This creation of yours is something which you ultimately become. Finally you come to realise that your creation is nothing other than your self-revelation.

True, there are as many missions as there are souls. But all missions fulfil themselves only after the souls have achieved some degree of perfection. The world is a divine play. Each participant plays a part in its success. The role of the servant is as important as that of the master. In the perfection of each individual part is the collective fulfilment. And at the same time, the individual fulfilment becomes perfect only when the individual has established his inseparable connection and realised his oneness with all human beings of the world.

You are one from the sole of your foot to the crown of your head. Yet at one place you are called ears, at another place you are called eyes. Each place in your body has a name of its own. Strangely enough, although they all are part of the same body, one cannot perform the action of another. Eyes see, but they cannot hear. Ears hear, but they cannot see. So the body, being one, also is many. Similarly, although God is one, He manifests Himself through many forms.

God tells us our mission. But we do not understand God's language, so He has to be His own interpreter. When others tell us about God, they can never tell us fully what God is. They misrepresent, and we misunderstand. God speaks in silence. Also, He interprets His message in silence. So also let us hear and understand God in silence.

Has your soul a special mission? Yes. Your mission is in the inmost recesses of your heart, and you have to find and fulfil it there. There can be no external way for you to fulfil your mission. The deer grows musk in his own body. He smells it and becomes enchanted, and tries to locate its source. He runs and runs, but he cannot find the source. In his endless search, he loses all his energy and finally he dies. But the source he was so desperately searching for was within himself. How could he find it elsewhere?

Such is the case with you. Your special mission — which is the fulfilment of your divinity — is not outside you, but within you. Search within. Meditate within. You will discover your mission.

Love

    The love that commands soulfully and the love that obeys unconditionally enjoy the selfsame Bliss of the Supreme.

HOW FAR ARE WE FROM REALISATION?

Avidyaya mrityum tirtha vidyaya amritam snute.
"By ignorance we cross through death, by knowledge we achieve Immortality." This is indeed a major realisation.

Realisation means the revelation of God in a human body. Realisation means that man himself is God.

Unfortunately, man is not alone. He has desire, and desire has tremendous power. Nevertheless, it fails to give him lasting joy and peace. Desire is finite. Desire is blind. It tries to bind man, who is boundless by birthright. God's Grace, which acts through man for God's full manifestation, is infinite.

Realisation springs from self-conquest. It grows in its oneness with God. It fulfils itself in embracing the finite and the Infinite.

We are seekers of the Supreme. What we need is absolute realisation. With a little realisation we can at most act like a cat. With absolute realisation we shall be able to threaten ignorance like a roaring lion.

The moment I say "my body," I separate myself from the body. This body undergoes infancy, childhood, adolescence, maturity and old age. It is not really me. The real "I" remains changeless always. When I say that I have grown fat or thin, I am speaking of the body that has grown fat or thin, and not the inner "I," which is eternal and immortal.

Realisation says that there are no such things as the bondage and freedom which we so often refer to in our day-to-day lives. What actually exists is consciousness — consciousness on various levels, consciousness enjoying itself in its varied manifestations. So long as we think that we are living in the bondage of ignorance, we are at liberty to feel that we can dwell in freedom as well, if we want to. If bondage makes us feel that the world is a field of suffering, then freedom can undoubtedly make us feel that the world is nothing but the blissful consciousness of the Brahman. But realisation makes us feel *Sarvam khalvidam Brahma.* "All that is extended is Brahman."

In order to realise what realisation is, we first have to love our inner Self. The second step is to love realisation itself. This is the love that awakens the soul. This is the love that illumines our consciousness. Love and you will be loved. Realise and you will be fulfilled.

Realisation is our inner lamp. If we keep the lamp burning, it will transmit to the world at large its radiant glow. We all, with no exceptions, have the power of self-realisation or, in

36

other words, God-realisation. To deny this truth is to deceive ourselves mercilessly.

We realise the Truth not only when joy fills our mind, but also when sorrow clouds our heart, when death welcomes us into its tenebrous breast, when Immortality places our existence in transformation's lap.

How far are we from Realisation? We can know the answer by the degree to which we have surrendered to God's Will. There is no other way to know it. Also we must know that every single day dawns with a new realisation. Life is a constant realisation to him whose inner eye is open.

Why do we want to realise God? We want to realise God because we consciously have made ourselves avenues through which the fruits of God-realisation can flow. Our very body is a divine machine; hence it needs oiling. Realisation is a divine lubricant, which does its work most effectively.

Realisation can be achieved by God's Grace, the Guru's grace and the seeker's aspiration. God's Grace is the rain. The Guru's grace is the seed. The seeker's aspiration is the act of cultivation. Lo, the bumper crop is Realisation!

Faith, Devotion, Surrender

Faith gives you what you have not: simplicity. Once you have simplicity, you will like it. Devotion gives you what you have not: purity. Once you have purity, you will love it. Surrender gives you what you have not: sincerity. Once you have sincerity, you will cherish it.

THE ROLE OF PURITY
IN THE SPIRITUAL LIFE

Purity! Purity! Purity! We love you. We want you. We need you. Stay in our thoughts! Stay in our actions! Stay in the breath of our life!

How to be pure? We can be pure by self-control. We can control our senses. It is unbelievably difficult, but it is not impossible.

"I shall control my senses. I shall conquer my passions." This approach cannot bring us what we actually want. The hungry lion that lives in our senses and the hungry tiger that lives in our passions will not leave us because of the mere repetition of the thought, "I shall control my senses and conquer my passions." This approach is of no avail.

What we must do is fix our mind on God. To our utter amazement, our lion and tiger, now tamed, will leave us of their own accord when they see that we have become too poor to feed them. But as a matter of fact, we have not become poor in the least. On the contrary, we have become infinitely stronger and richer, for God's Will energizes our body, mind and heart. To fix our body, mind and heart on the Divine is the right approach. The closer we are to the Light, the farther we are from the darkness.

39

Purity does not come all at once. It takes time. We must dive deep and lose ourselves with implicit faith in contemplation of God. We need not go to Purity. Purity will come to us. And Purity does not come alone. It brings an ever-lasting Joy with it. This divine Joy is the sole purpose of our life. God reveals Himself fully and manifests Himself unreservedly only when we have this inner Joy.

The world gives us desires. God gives us prayers. The world gives us bondage. God gives us freedom: freedom from limitations, freedom from ignorance.

We are the player. We can play either football or cricket. We have a free choice. Similarly, it is we who can choose either purity or impurity to play with. The player is the master of the game, and not vice versa.

The easiest and most effective way to have purity is to repeat a *mantra*. A *mantra* is a seed-sound. A *mantra* is a dynamic power in the form of a vibrant sound.

Now let us know what *japa* is. *Japa* is the repetition of a *mantra*. You want purity, don't you? Then right now, repeat the name of God five hundred times. This is our *mantra*. Let us all do it.

(The seekers joined Sri Chinmoy in repeating the mantra.)

Thank you. We are successful. Now every day please increase the number by one hundred.

That is to say, tomorrow you will repeat the name of God six hundred times, and the day after, seven hundred. One week from today my calculation says that you will repeat the name of God twelve hundred times. From that day please start decreasing the number daily by one hundred until you again reach five hundred. Please continue this exercise, week by week, just for a month. Whether you want to change your name or not, the world will give you a new name. It will call you by the name Purity. Your inner ear will make you hear it. It will surpass your fondest imagination.

Let nothing perturb us. Let our body's impurity remind us of our heart's spontaneous Purity. Let our outer finite thoughts remind us of our inner infinite Will. Let our mind's teeming imperfections remind us of our soul's limitless Perfection.

The present-day world is full of impurity. It seems that purity is a currency from another world. It is hard to obtain this purity, but once we get it, peace is ours, success is ours.

Let us face the world. Let us take life as it comes. Our Inner Pilot is constantly vigilant. The undercurrents of our inner and spiritual life will always flow on unnoticed, unobstructed, unafraid.

God may be unknown but He is not unknowable. Our prayers and meditation lead us to that unknown. Freedom we cry for. But strangely enough, we are not aware of the fact that we already have within us immense freedom. Look!

Without any difficulty, we can forget God. We can ignore Him and we can even deny Him. But God's Compassion says, "My children, no matter what you do or say, My Heart shall never abandon you. I want you. I need you."

The mother holds the hand of the child. But it is the child who has to walk, and he does so. Neither the one who is dragged nor the one who drags can be happy. Likewise, God says, "My divine children, in your inner life, I give you inspiration. It is you who have to aspire with the purest heart to reach the Golden Beyond."

TWO SECRETS:
REINCARNATION AND EVOLUTION

To understand the secrets of reincarnation, evolution and transformation we must first understand the most significant secret of all: the secret of *karma*.

Karma is a Sanskrit word which means action. The heart can perform it; the mind can perform it; the body can perform it.

There are three kinds of *karma: Sanchita karma, Prarabdha karma* and *Agami karma*.

Sanchita means amassed. We wait consciously or unconsciously for the fruit of *karma* that we have sown by our past thoughts, words, deeds and volitions. *Sanchita karma* is an accumulation of acts done in some past life or in this life, whose results have not yet been worked out, whose effects have not yet been produced.

Prarabdha karma is fate or destiny as the result of acts done in any former birth. The karmic effects have begun, but they are not yet finished and necessitate rebirth for completion. *Prarabdha karma* is that part of *Sanchita karma* which has started bearing fruit. We begin reaping in this life the fruit of our past *karma,* and at the same time we sow new seeds for future reaping.

Agami means future or approaching. *Agami karma* can be done only after one has attained spiritual perfection, when one is bound neither by the lure of birth nor by the snares of death. One acts then with a view to helping humanity. To fulfil the Divine here on earth, the liberated soul in this case plays a significant role in the Divine Play which has no beginning, no ending.

We know that there is some Being whom we call God. We know that there is something which we call the soul. It was the great American philosopher, Emerson, who said: "God is an infinite circle whose centre is everywhere, but whose circumference is nowhere." We can say definitely that this centre is man's soul.

The soul is an eternal entity. What is its connection with reincarnation? One could write endless pages on reincarnation, that formidable concept which is so widely spoken about and just as widely disbelieved. Let us try to understand, in one short sentence, the essence of the matter. Reincarnation is the process by which the soul evolves; it exists for the growth and development of the soul.

We all know Charles Darwin's theory of evolution of species. It is the change in the physical organism from lower to higher, or from simpler to more complex. Spiritual evolution runs parallel to physical evolution. The soul exists in all beings. True, it is divine and immortal. But it has its own urge to be more complete, more fulfilling and more divine. Hence, in the process of its evolution, it has to pass from the least perfect body to the most perfect body. At each stage, it takes into itself the real value of all its earthly experiences. Thus the soul grows, enriching itself, making its divinity more integral, more harmonious and more perfect.

Reincarnation tells us that we have not come from nothing. Our present condition is the result of what we have made ourselves from our past. We are the consequence of our past incarnations.

"Many births have been left behind by me and by thee, O Arjuna! All of them I know, but thou knowest not thine." So said the divine Sri Krishna to the yet unrealised Arjuna.

Evolution is the hyphen between what was and what shall be. I am a man. I must know that not only was I my father, but also shall I be my son. Problems I had. You had. He had. No exceptions! We faced them. We face them even today. But we shall solve them unmistakably.

The Permanent Law of God

To forget the dark futility of blind igno-rance is the permanent Law of God. To for-give the scorching heat of human pride is the permanent Law of God. To see oneself always with a smiling face and an adaman-tine will is the permanent Law of God.

WHAT IS THE AIM OF LIFE?

The aim of life is to become conscious of the Supreme Reality. The aim of life is to be the conscious expression of the Eternal Being.

Life is evolution. Evolution is the unfoldment from within. Each life is a world in itself. Indeed, each life is a microcosm. Whatever breathes in the vast universe also breathes in each individual life.

There are two lives: the inner and the outer. The outer life speaks about its principles and then tries to act. It professes in season and out of season, but it practises very little of what it professes. The inner life does not speak. It acts. Its spontaneous action is the conscious manifestation of God.

Our life has two realities: exoteric and esoteric. The exoteric reality deals with the outer world. The outer reality tries to fulfil itself by feeding desires and stimulating passions. The esoteric or inner reality finds fulfilment in the control of passions and the conquest of desires, in swimming in the vast sea of Liberation.

Life is existence. The ordinary existence comes from a deeper Existence. Existence cannot come from non-existence. Life comes from God. Life is God. Two things we should do: we should study life most devotedly and live life most divinely.

Two things we must have: imagination and inspiration. A life with no imagination is a life of imprisonment. With the wings of imagination, we must try to fly into the Beyond. A life with no inspiration is a life of stagnation. With the dynamism of ceaseless inspiration, we shall give new meaning to life and immortalize life.

The aim of life is to realise God. Realisation can never come to the individual who is inactive. We have to strive for Realisation. We have to pay the price for it. There is no alternative. One thing of paramount importance: by telling others that you are a realised soul, you may convince others, you may even deceive your own heart, but you cannot deceive God.

For God-Realisation, the first requisite is peace. Peace is based on love: love for humanity and love for God. Peace is also founded on non-attachment. No thirst for gain, no fear of loss, lo! peace is yours. Peace is also based on renunciation. This renunciation is not the renunciation of worldly possessions, but of limitation and ignorance. That peace is the true Peace which is not affected by the roaring of the world, outer or inner.

When you have that divine Peace, Realisation cannot help knocking at your heart's door. To be more accurate, the Lotus of Realisation will start blooming in your heart, petal by petal.

For God-Realisation, temples, churches and synagogues are not obligatory. Neither is the tapestry of scriptures and sermons required. What is imperative is meditation. This meditation will make you realise God the Infinite within your soul, heart, mind and body.

The aim of life is to live a divine life. We are living in this world. We know that man does not live by bread alone. He needs the soul in order to live in the world of God's Reality. The soul alone has the capacity to see and feel the known and the Unknown, the existent and the non-existent, the dream of the past, the achievement of the present and the hope of the future.

Let us accept the inner life, the spiritual life. Mistakes in our journey are inevitable. Success without endeavour is impossibility itself. No work, no progress. Experience we must welcome, for we can learn nothing without experience. The experience may be either encouraging or discouraging. But it is experience that makes us a real being, that shows us the true meaning of our very existence.

Let us all be truly spiritual. Let us realise God through our constant communion with Him. We need not have any particular time or place for our meditation. We must transcend the necessity of time and space. When we go deep within, we feel that one moment cannot be separated from another, that one place cannot be separated from another. Let us aspire to live in the Eternal Now of God-Realisation, in the Eternal Now of God's Dream and Reality. This

Dream is the Dream of ever-surpassing Transcendence. This Reality is the Reality of ever-blossoming Revelation.

WHAT IS SPIRITUALITY?

Spirituality is the universality of Truth, Light and Bliss. Spirituality is the conscious necessity for God. Spirituality is the constant opportunity to realise and prove that we all can be as great as God.

God is Delight. Delight is the breath of the soul. God does not want to see the face of sorrow. God will give us infinitude the moment we are ready to offer Him just one flash of our soul's delight.

Sorrowful is the world. We are responsible for it. Our feelings of self-interest and self-importance are fully responsible for it. The individual consciousness must expand. Man needs inspiration. Man needs action. Spirituality needs man. Spirituality needs absolute fulfilment. Spirituality has the inner eye that links every condition of life with inner certitude.

Man can make and unmake his outer conditions by his spiritual thoughts. He who carries God in his thoughts and actions, to him alone is God a living Reality.

Spirituality has a secret key to open the Door of the Divine. This key is meditation. Meditation simplifies our outer life and energizes our inner life. Meditation gives us a natural and spontaneous life. This life becomes so natural and spontaneous that we cannot breathe without the consciousness of our divinity.

Meditation is a divine gift. It is the direct approach, for it leads the aspirant to the One from whom he has descended. Meditation tells us that our human life is a secret and sacred thing, and it affirms our divine heritage. Meditation gives us a new eye to see God, a new ear to hear the Voice of God and a new heart to feel the Presence of God.

The spiritual life is not a bed of roses; neither is it a bed of thorns. It is a bed of reality and inevitability. In my spiritual life, I see the role of the devil and the role of my Lord. If the devil has temptation, my Lord has Guidance. If the devil has opposition, my Lord has Help. If the devil has punishment, my Lord has Compassion. If the devil takes me to hell, my Lord takes me to Heaven. If the devil has death for me, my Lord has Immortality for me.

Out of the fulness of our heart, and with tears flooding our eyes, we must pray to God. We must pitch our aim as high as God-realisation, for that is the sole aim of our earthly existence. Sri Ramakrishna says: "He is born to no purpose who, having the rare privilege of being born a man, is unable to realise God in this life."

Science has achieved marvels. Nevertheless, its range of vision is limited. There are worlds beyond the senses; there are hidden mysteries.

Science has no access to these worlds; science can never solve these mysteries. But a spiritual figure with his inner vision can easily enter into these worlds and fathom these mysteries. Yet a spiritual figure is a real idealist who does not build castles in the air, but rather has his feet firmly planted on the ground.

Spirituality is not merely tolerance. It is not even acceptance. It is the feeling of universal oneness. In our spiritual life, we look upon the Divine, not only in terms of our own God, but in terms of everybody's God. Our spiritual life firmly and securely establishes the basis of unity in diversity.

Spirituality is not mere hospitality to others' faith in God. It is the absolute recognition and acceptance of their faith in God as one's own. Difficult, but not impossible, for this has been the experience and practice of all spiritual Masters of all times.

"Truth" has been the problem of problems in every age. Truth lives in experience. Truth, in its outer aspect, is sincerity, truthfulness and integrity. Truth, in its inner and spiritual aspect, is the vision of God, the realisation of God and the manifestation of God. That which eternally breathes is Truth. Soul-stirring is the cry of our Upanishadic seers: *Satyam eva jayate nanritam:* "Truth alone triumphs, and not untruth." Blessed is India to have this as her motto, her life-breath, her far-flung message of universal divinity.

Spirituality is not to be found in books.

Even if we squeeze a book, we will get no spirituality. If we want to be spiritual, we have to grow from within. Thoughts and ideas precede books. The mind arouses thoughts and ideas from their slumber. Spirituality awakens the mind. A spiritual man is he who listens to the dictates of his soul, and whom fear cannot torture. The opinions of the world are too weak to torment his mind and heart. This truth he knows, feels and embodies.

Finally, I have an open secret for those who want to launch into the spiritual life. The open secret is this: you can change your life. You need not wait years or even months for this change. It begins the moment you dive into the sea of spirituality. Try to live the life of spiritual discipline for a day, a single day! You are bound to succeed.

WHAT IS YOGA?

What is Yoga? Yoga is the language of God. If we wish to speak to God, we have to learn His language.

What is Yoga? Yoga is that which discloses God's secret. If we wish to know God's secret, we have to launch into the path of Yoga.

What is Yoga? Yoga is the Breath of God. If we wish to see through God's Eye and feel through His Heart, if we wish to live in God's Dream and know God's Reality, if we wish to possess the Breath of God, and finally if we wish to become God Himself, Yoga will beckon us.

Yoga is union. It is the union of the individual soul with the Supreme Self. Yoga is the spiritual science that teaches us how the Ultimate Reality can be realised in life itself.

What we have to do is accept life and fulfil the Divine in ourselves here on earth. This can be effectuated only by transcending our human limitations.

Yoga tells us how far we have progressed in relation to God-realisation. It also tells us about our destined role in God's cosmic Drama. The final word of Yoga is that each human soul is a divine representative of God on earth.

Now let us focus our attention on the practical aspect of Yoga. There are various kinds of Yoga: *Karma Yoga*, the path of action; *Bhakti Yoga,* the path of love and devotion; and *Jnana Yoga,* the path of knowledge. These three are considered to be the most important kinds of Yoga. There are other significant types of Yoga, but they are either branches of these three or types closely related to them.

These three serve as the three main gates to God's Palace. If we want to see and feel God in the sweetest and most intimate way, then we have to practise *Bhakti Yoga.* If we want to realise God in humanity through our selfless service, then we have to practise *Karma Yoga.* If we want to realise the wisdom and glories of God's transcendental Self, then we have to practise *Jnana Yoga.*

One thing is certain. These three paths lead us to Self-realisation in God-realisation and God-realisation in Self-realisation.

BHAKTI YOGA, KARMA YOGA
AND JNANA YOGA

BHAKTI YOGA

Ask a man to speak about God and he will speak
endlessly. Ask a Bhakta to speak about God and
he will say only two things: God is all Affection,
God is all Sweetness. The Bhakta even goes one
step further. He says, "I can try to live without
bread, but never can I live without my Lord's
Grace."

A Bhakta's prayer is very simple: "O my
Lord God, do enter into my life with Thine Eye
of Protection and with Thy Heart of Compassion." This prayer is the quickest way to knock
at God's Door and also the easiest way to see
God open the Door.

A Karma yogin and a Jnana yogin may suffer
a moment of doubt about God's existence. But
a Bhakta has no suffering of that type. To him,
the existence of God is an axiomatic truth. More
than that, it is his heart's spontaneous feeling.
But alas, he too has to undergo a kind of suffering. His is the suffering of separation from his
Beloved. With the tears of his heart's devotion,

57

he cries to re-establish his sweetest union with God.

The reasoning mind does not charm the Bhakta devotee. The hard facts of life fail to draw his attention, let alone absorb him. He wants to live constantly in a God-intoxicated realm.

A devotee feels that when he walks toward God, God runs toward him. A devotee feels that when he thinks of God for a second, God cries for him for an hour. A devotee feels that when he goes to God with a drop of his love to quench God's ceaseless thirst, God enfolds him in the sea of His ambrosial Love.

The relation between a devotee and God can only be felt, never described. Poor God thinks that no man on earth can ever capture Him, for He is priceless and invaluable. Alas, He has forgotten that He has already granted devotion to His Bhakta. To His greatest surprise, to His deepest joy, His devotee's surrendered devotion is able to capture Him.

There are people who mock the Bhakta. They say that a Bhakta's God is nothing but a personal God, an infinite God with form, a glorified human being. To them I say, "Why should a Bhakta not feel thus?" A Bhakta sincerely feels that he is a tiny drop and that God is the infinite Ocean. He feels that his body is an infinitesimal portion of God the boundless Whole. A devotee thinks of a God and prays to a God in his own image. And he is absolutely right to do so. Just enter into a cat's consciousness and you will see that its idea of an omnipotent Being takes the form of a cat — only in a gigantic form. Just enter into the consciousness of a flower and you will see that the flower's idea of something infinitely more beautiful than itself takes the image of a flower.

The Bhakta does the same. He knows that he is a human being and he feels that his God should be human in every sense of the term. The only difference, he feels, is that he is a limited human being and God is a limitless human Being.

To a devotee, God is at once blissful and merciful. His heart's joy makes him feel that God is blissful and his heart's pangs make him feel that God is merciful.

A bird sings. A man sings. God too sings. He sings His sweetest songs of Infinity, Eternity and Immortality through the heart of His Bhakta.

KARMA YOGA

Karma Yoga is desireless action undertaken for the sake of the Supreme. *Karma Yoga* is man's genuine acceptance of his earthly existence. *Karma Yoga* is man's dauntless march across the battlefield of life.

Karma Yoga does not see eye to eye with those who hold that the activities of human life are of no importance. *Karma Yoga* claims that life is a divine opportunity for serving God. This particular Yoga is not only the Yoga of physical action; it includes the aspirant's moral and inner life as well.

Those who follow this path pray for a strong and perfect body. They also pray for a long life. This long life is not a mere prolongation of life in terms of years. It is a life that longs for the descent of the divine Truth, Light and Power into the material plane. The Karma yogins are the real heroes on the earthly scene, and theirs is the divinely triumphant victory.

A Karma yogin is a perfect stranger to the waves of disappointment and despair in human life. What he sees in life and its activities is a divine purpose. He feels himself to be the hyphen between earthly duties and heavenly responsibilities. He has many weapons to conquer the world, but his detachment is the most powerful. His detachment defies both the crushing blows of failure and the ego-gratifying surges of success. His detachment is far beyond both the snares of the world's excruciating pangs and the embrace of the world's throbbing joy.

Many sincere aspirants feel that the devotional feelings of a Bhakta and the penetrating eye of a Jnani have no place in *Karma Yoga*. Here they are quite mistaken. A true Karma yogin is he whose heart has implicit faith in God, whose mind has a constant awareness of God and whose body has a genuine love for God in humanity.

It is easy for a Bhakta to forget the world, and for a Jnani to ignore the world. But a Karma yogin's destiny is otherwise. God wants him to live in the world, live with the world and live for the world.

JNANA YOGA

God has three eyes. Their names are *Bhakti, Karma* and *Jnana. Bhakti* wants to live in its Father's most intimate Truth. *Karma* wants to live in its Father's all-pervading universal Truth. *Jnana* wants to live in its Father's transcendental Truth.

The man of devotion needs God's protection. The man of action needs God's guidance. The man of knowledge needs God's instruction.

The Bhakta's faith in God and the Karma yogin's love for humanity do not interest a Jnana yogin, much less inspire him. He wants nothing but the mind. With his mental power he strives for the personal experience of the highest Truth. He thinks of God as the Fount of Knowledge. He feels that it is through his mind that he will attain his Goal. At the beginning of his path, he feels that nothing is as important as the fulfilment of the mind. Eventually he comes to realise that he must transcend the mind if he wishes to live in the Supreme Knowledge.

Life is a mystery. So is death. A Jnana yogin wants to fathom these two apparently insoluble mysteries of God's creation. He also wants to

61

transcend both life and death and abide in the Heart of the Supreme Reality.

Man lives in the sense world. He does not know whether this world is real or unreal. An ordinary man is satisfied with his own existence. He has neither the thinking capacity nor the sincere interest to enter into the deeper meaning of life. He wants to escape the problems of life and death. Unfortunately, there is no escape. He has to swim in the sea of ignorance. A Jnana yogin alone can teach him how to swim across the sea of ignorance and enter the Sea of Knowledge and Light.

A Jnana yogin declares: *Neti, neti.* "Not this, not this." What does he mean? He means that there is a higher world than this sense-world, a higher truth than this earthbound truth. He says, in a sense, that there are two opposing parties. One party consists of falsehood, ignorance and death. The other party consists of Truth, Knowledge and Immortality. While uttering "*Neti, neti*" he asks man to reject falsehood and accept Truth, reject ignorance and accept Knowledge, reject death and accept Immortality.

WHAT IS GOD'S PLAN?

What is God's plan? This question is often raised and discussed. Strangely enough, the very idea of God's plan attracts the attention, not only of those who believe in God, but also of those who deny God's existence.

Has God a plan? No, never! Making a plan means drawing up an estimate of work to be done in the future. It is the temptation of success that often inspires us to throw ourselves into activities. We want to grow into the success of the future. Hence, plans do help us to some extent. But God needs no plan. To Him, the vision of the Future is not a thing to be fulfilled, but a thing that already abides, nay, looms large in the giant breast of the present.

The world has ever been charmed by movement, here, there and everywhere. The waning of enthusiastic movement is the downfall of human life. Each movement has to undergo ups and downs before it reaches its goal. Movement is the outer expression of an inner urge. This inner urge is the representative of God's Will in a human body seeking to play with the Beyond and to awaken the Infinite in the finite.

God has no plan. Neither does He need one. He is not a mental being who cannot think of the future without a plan. What God is, is Delight. What God wants us to have is Delight. We can have it only by turning all that we have and all that we are towards the Supreme Reality.

We must think of God's existence first, and then, if we must, we may think of God's plan. Does God exist? Where is the proof? Our very heart is the proof. Constantly our heart demands or begs of us to see God everywhere and in everything. With the aspiration of our heart, God's existence can be felt. With the aspiration of our heart we can see that God's Heaven, which is Silence, and God's earth, which is Power, are not only interdependent, but also complementary smiles of God's eternal Reality.

Some people say that the world has come into existence from a plan made by God. They see that the world is full of suffering and imperfection and feel that they could have made a better world if they had been given a chance. To them I say, "Who prevents you? It is you who have to cultivate the soil in order to grow a bumper crop of perfection and satisfaction."

Much have we learned from suffering and imperfection. What we need now is Delight and Perfection. We cannot have these two divine qualities by finding fault with a plan that we have thrust upon God. We can have Delight and Perfection only by living in God's Consciousness. There is no other way.

Man's interpretation of suffering and imperfection is based on his preconceived mental ideas and notions. God's interpretation is founded on His direct Vision in its absolute and ultimate Reality. Man's interpretation needs justification. But God's interpretation does not need any justification, for He is at once the Truth embodied and the Truth revealed.

Similarly, a spiritual man looks at God from a different angle than does an ordinary man. He feels that God has and is everything, manifest and unmanifest. His God is in the eternal process of ever-progressing Perfection. An ordinary man, however, feels that God has yet to achieve something to transform the world.

God is a child, an eternal divine Child. How can a child have a plan? Impossible! Just as a human child plays with his dolls, dressing and fondling them, so God, the divine Child, does the same with His dolls, the human instruments. But being the divine Child, God, whatever He does, He does consciously, significantly and divinely.

Man's unconscious, semi-conscious, conscious and spiritually conscious plans and God's self-revealing manifestations are inseparable. The Supreme Secret is that man's plans are always united with the Breath of the Supreme. Man has to know this. Nothing further is there to know. Man has to feel this. Nothing deeper is there to feel. Man has to realise this. Nothing higher is there to realise.

A Prayer

When morning clears, I pray to God to inspire me, I pray to God to aspire within me, I pray to God to concentrate on me, I pray to God to meditate for me.

PART TWO:

QUESTIONS AND ANSWERS

Renunciation

No renunciation can be commanded.
No renunciation can be demanded.
Renunciation has to grow from within.
Renunciation has to flow from without.
Man renounces the futility of his igno-
rance-night.
God announces man, Infinity's Light.

QUESTIONS AND ANSWERS
ON THE INNER LIFE

1.

How can one reconcile America's inner decay and crassness with her evolving spiritual awareness?

Your question is·at once extremely interesting and thought-provoking. It is a question about which one could say much. I wish to reflect on it, not from the sociological viewpoint, but from the spiritual viewpoint, which is not so well understood.

America's inner decay is, to me, not so grave nor so vital as you feel it to be. I take it to be a battle between darkness and Light. When we consciously open ourselves to the Light, inevitably all our unconscious weaknesses and limitations come forward to bar the way. The more the Light beckons us, the stronger become our unruly, undivine and unconscious parts. This is an inescapable spiritual law, which we can see operating in the individual as well as in the collectivity. Before proceeding to your question about America, let me explain why this law exists.

Ignorance has always ruled the earth, and even now it continues to dominate the earth-consciousness. The material world has not consciously aspired for its own inner fulfilment, which is part of a destined integral spiritual fulfilment of humanity. Darkness has always been the master. It does not want a higher force to take its place, so it fights with all its power to perpetuate its rule. And so, when the divine force succeeds in making an opening in a certain area of the earth-consciousness and is rewarded with a renewed aspiration, the undivine forces also intensify their efforts, creating values and ideas which are utterly empty of any higher truth. This eternal battle between darkness and Light becomes even more intense when a new and higher cycle is about to begin in the evolution of mankind, which is the case today.

These are the primary reasons for your feeling that a yawning chasm exists between America's high aspiration and ideals on the one hand, and some of her unlit actions and values on the other. Her evolving spiritual awareness and her hasty outer movements are not quite in collaboration with each other; they are not helping one another. Until the Light dawns fully, the true seeking cannot come forward wholeheartedly; hence, the values leading to integral spiritual progress are not much in evidence.

America, moreover, is a young nation. It does not want to walk; it wants to run as fast as possible in order to breast the tape first. You know that while running at top speed there is every possibility of stumbling or running off the track. Nevertheless, with America's sincere and dynamic urge for progress, her present gropings and wanderings will pale into insignificance as we vision the promise and possibilities of her future fulfilment.

2.

Do you not feel that national boundaries, economic disparity and religious dogma divide human beings into different camps, creating unspiritual environments and making peace, for an individual as well as for a nation, a distant star?

I do strongly feel that these national boundaries and so forth are really impairing the growth of our evolving human consciousness. But it is the clarification of the individual's mind and spirit that must precede the awakening of our social institutions such as churches and governments. It is the spiritual and mental elite who can infuse the general mass with their illumining light. As we know, the policies of institutions and nations are usually embodiments of the general consciousness. These policies can be influenced considerably by enlightened individuals. Mother India in particular has not lacked in such enlightened souls, nor does she lack them now.

It is only a matter of time until time itself will create an opening so the spiritual consciousness may permeate the individual and his society. On our part, a conscious spiritual effort has to be made so that the higher forces from above can come down and touch the very depths of our seeking hearts. When this occurs, the gap that we now see between our aspiration and its fulfilment in society will no longer exist.

3.

I would frankly like to know what India's spirituality has ever done for her. How is it that in spite of her yogis and saints, she is still a poor and backward country?

First, we must understand what has brought this situation about. In ancient India, the material life was not renounced. People in those days aspired for a synthesis of Matter and Spirit, and to some extent they were successful in achieving it. But there is a great gulf between that hoary past and the present.

In the later periods of India's history, the saints and seers came to feel that the material life and the spiritual life could never go together, that they had to renounce the outer life in order to attain to God. Hence, the external life was neglected. This led to foreign conquests and many other troubles. Even today, the attitude that material prosperity and beauty should be negated is very common in India. This accounts for much of her continued poverty.

But at present there are spiritual giants in India who feel that God should be realised in His totality, that Creator and creation are one and inseparable. They advocate the acceptance of life, the real need for both progress and perfection in all spheres of human existence. This new approach is widely accepted in modern India.

India may be poverty-stricken today, but she will progress quickly by virtue of her new awareness and her new aspiration. She has not only magnanimity of heart but also the power to bring her soul's strength to the fore and use it to solve all her problems.

4.

Could you please tell me why people in India worship so many gods and goddesses and not one?

Could you please tell me why you worship the Father, the Son, the Holy Ghost and so many angels and saints? We in India have many gods and goddesses. As a matter of fact, we feel that each individual must have a god of his own, that each man must have his own process of realising God.

Indeed, these gods and goddesses are simply different manifestations of the Sole Absolute. Each deity embodies a particular aspect or quality of the Supreme. Our inability to recognize the all-embracing universal Harmony in all these different aspects gives rise to our misunderstandings and disputes. The moment we realise the universal Spirit, the impersonal One, we can be in perfect harmony with all the different beliefs.

Then we can see the truth behind the conception of the various gods and goddesses.

5.

The caste system is absolutely bad. Why do you have it? Can you say even one word in favour of it?

Well, I must take exception to your comment and tell you that in this world there is nothing absolutely bad. The caste system has served and even now continues to serve a certain purpose. In spite of all its degenerations, it has been a system that has united the different parts of society. If we try to see it as a system uniting people instead of dividing them, we will better understand the value that it has had for thousands of years. Society was conceived as a great family. Each group worked to make it function harmoniously. In a family, one brother may be a spiritual teacher, another an executive, a third a merchant and the fourth a farmer. Each one helps the family in his own way at the time of need. It is their combined knowledge and harmonious co-operation which create a real unity in their family life. So was it originally with the caste system. Each group had responsibilities and duties. Each group worked for the good of the whole. The important thing is how this system was utilized. In its ideal form the caste system has much truth and value, but the wrong attitudes which have entered into it through human ignorance require that the present system be supplanted with something more suited to a modern and advanced society.

6.

If an Indian living here marries an American girl, will his parents accept them when they go to India?

It depends entirely on the parents. If they are orthodox and conservative, they may not accept them. But if the parents are liberal in their ideas and cherish broad ideals, if they value the link between East and West, then they will gladly accept their son and daughter-in-law. From the spiritual point of view, in God's Light, it is not race or religion, but the true fulfilment of two human souls in union that is of supreme importance.

7.

Is it true that some people in India can walk on fire? Doesn't it scare you or astonish you?

I have twice had the opportunity to witness such a performance. I was not afraid because fortunately I was not one of the performers. And I was not astonished because I was aware of the power of faith. They had a tremendous faith in Govinda (Lord Krishna). Chanting the name of Govinda with intense devotion, they walked unscathed over the fire.

8.

In India, the wives surrender to their husbands. Why do they not care for their own individuality?

I hope that you know the meaning of surrender. In real surrender, we do not lose our individuality. On the contrary, we enlarge it. For example, when we surrender ourselves absolutely to God, we become one with God in our adoration for Him. His Power is then added to ours. Surrender is entirely voluntary. Submitting out of fear, to someone more powerful than ourselves, is not surrender. True surrender is a great strength which fulfils itself when it becomes one with the object of its adoration. In India, women cheerfully and unreservedly surrender their very existence to their husbands and get the real joy of true union.

9.

You have explained to us what the supreme surrender is. Now I would like to know from you what the supreme sacrifice is.

My young friend, it gives me great pleasure to hear your question. The supreme sacrifice is self-sacrifice for a noble cause. To fulfil God, if necessity demands, you may have to embrace death. To uplift humanity, if necessity demands, you may have to forego your own immortality.

The supreme sacrifice is this. Let us try. It is worth aspiring for.

10.

If man, when dissatisfied with the world, escapes the world and seeks out higher planes of existence, how will humanity ever be able to establish peace and happiness on earth?

Your question shows a remarkable sense of spiritual values. Granted, the world is all imperfection. Life stands as a huge question. Evil is seen everywhere. These are the problems that we face every day. Moreover, the more spiritually advanced a man is, the greater is his suffering, due to the present conditions of the world. He sees the disease, he feels the disease, but he has no proper medicine. Even if he has a remedy, it is not enough to cure all earthly ailments. So he often feels that his fight will be of no avail and therefore takes the easier path, the path of escape into the Bliss of the higher planes.

But this can never be the case with a divine warrior. He will fight until the victory is won. Now what do we mean by his "victory"? It is the establishment of the Kingdom of God here on earth and not in some higher world. As he knows that the Divine is omnipresent, he seeks to reveal Him in everyday life. If we are not satisfied with the world as it is, that is no reason for leaving it. On the contrary, we should try to change it — physically or intellectually or spiritually, depending on our own development and capacities.

God is perfect Perfection. This Perfection can be achieved only when there is an inseparable union between Matter and Spirit, between the outer and the inner Life.

11.

My wife, who is otherwise the most reasonable of beings, insists that all religious beliefs are delusions brought about by existential anxiety. Most people find the thought unbearable that there is no meaning in life except for the biological and rational fact of life itself. But this, she feels, should satisfy anybody. The fact of death, she believes, is to be similarly faced as a biological reality. It is an old theory, which I realise can neither be proved or disproved at an intellectual level.

The ultimate truth concerning life and death can never be adequately explained or expressed. It can only be felt by the aspirant and known by the realised soul. I concur fully with you that this idea, as well as that expressed by your wife, cannot be verified intellectually. However, what your wife feels about life and death cannot be proven to be any more true than what you feel about them.

Human memory is not the first and last word in reality. If, at the age of eighty, I fail to recollect any incidents in my life that took place before I reached the age of four, it does not mean that I did not exist before that. Just as a series of years passes by as we go from the age of four to eighty, so is there a series of lives which connects the present with the distant past and projects itself into the imminent future.

Then, too, there is something beyond the comprehension of our limited body-consciousness. Even while a man is grossly involved in the most ordinary physical activities, he may feel within himself, at times, some strange truths. These are usually unfamiliar and greatly elevating. These truths come from a higher or deeper world, from a different plane of consciousness, and they knock at his mental door. Thus he possesses and is possessed by forces beyond his ordinary awareness.

It is when we put ourselves in tune with these higher forces — indeed, with the universal harmony — that life ceases to be unbearable. I entirely agree with your wife's view that when a person sees no meaning in life, no goal or purpose, this attitude, nay the life itself, becomes intolerable. However, regarding religious beliefs, I wish to place before her an analogy:

I am now living in a Brooklyn apartment. If a child calls on me and asks, "Is there a place called Cologne?" I shall reply, "Certainly, my child, it is in West Germany." Suppose he says, "You must prove it to me!" Now how can I prove it to him, apart from showing him maps and photos? I can only tell him that I have personally visited Cologne and that there are millions of others who have also done so. His doubt cannot negate the existence of the city.

Similarly, those who have realised God fully have every right to tell us that there is a God. Just because we have not realised Him ourselves, we cannot deny His existence. Just as the child has to satisfy his physical eyes by going to Cologne, we can only prove to ourselves the reality of God by seeing Him. And this quest for God gives to an otherwise purposeless life an unparalleled meaning and direction.

12.

I believe that love is always the same, whether human or divine. Is this true?

No, my young friend, human love and divine Love are two completely different things. If I give you fifteen cents and you give me a piece of candy, that is called human love. In divine Love, you don't wait for my fifteen cents. You give me the piece of candy cheerfully of your own accord. Divine Love is sacrifice, and in this sacrifice we are fulfilling God's Will, consciously or unconsciously. In human love, we display the buyer's and the seller's love, which is synonymous with self-interest. Mind you, I am not saying that human beings cannot express divine Love. They can and sometimes do. But consistent divine Love is, at present, rare in human beings.

13

You have been speaking of faith. Could you make it a bit easier for me to understand this concept?

Let me try. First of all, faith is not credulity or blind belief. It does not mean that you must constantly believe in the impossible. No, that is not faith. Faith is a spontaneous feeling. It does not care for human justification. It is the eye that visions the future and is always in tune with a higher truth. The door of faith is always open to the Truth-Beyond and, by virtue of faith, we transcend ourselves.

14.

How may we strengthen our inner faith in God when we are beset with discouragements in our daily life?

Please try to feel from now on that there is Somebody around you who does not want anything from you except joy. There is Somebody who wants you always to swim in the Sea of Joy and Delight. If you can remain in joy — I don't mean the outer joy of going here and there, mixing with people, buying material things — but if you can have real joy and inner fulfilment, then you will automatically have faith in God.

When we are worried, or are afraid of something, we immediately try to create a kind of self-imposed faith in God. This is not true faith. When we are in danger, we say, "God, save me, save me!" But we say this only to avert danger. This is an escape. This kind of faith does not last. Everything is inside a person, both joy and fulfilment. But who is the possessor of this inner fulfilment? It is God. We are just His devoted instruments. When we feel spontaneous inner joy as part and parcel of our life, and we feel its source, we can then have faith in God, the possessor of infinite Joy. From now on, please try to feel your own inner joy, and faith will come to you spontaneously. In regard to your outer frustrations, please do not try to unite them with your inner joy. Please separate your inner joy from the outer happenings. Only then will you be able to strengthen your faith in God.

15.

I have studied a good many scriptures. I also indulge in preaching about spirituality, religion, the inner life and so forth. But personally, I feel a barren desert within me. I get no satisfaction at all from what I am doing. I feel I am wasting my own precious time and that of others. Could you possibly enlighten me regarding this?

I fully sympathize with you. You are not alone. There are a good many human souls sailing in the same boat. The study of books and scriptures can give us information to quote, and a certain understanding. It can give us, at most, inspiration, but nothing more. By borrowing others' ideas, we can never be truly enlightened in our inner life. It is by studying the eternal book of Truth within us, by listening constantly to the Voice of the inner Self, that we can become spiritually illumined. It is then that we will find joy in our outer life. We must see God first, and then we can become Godlike. If we want to be truly Godlike, our talking must give way to becoming. Let me tell you a true story.

In a certain village in Bengal, India, a rich man's servant went to his master's house every day by crossing a river in a ferry boat. One day there was a violent storm. The ferry could not cross the raging river and the servant, who was forced to go many miles out of his way to a foot bridge, was late in arriving. His master was furious. "You fool," he shouted, "if you utter Krishna's name three times, you will see that you don't need a boat. You will be able to walk across the river!"

That afternoon, as the storm showed no signs of abating, the poor servant was threatened with the same situation. But, in his simple faith, he obeyed his master's instructions. From the very depths of his heart he uttered the name of Krishna. Lo, the miracle of miracles! He felt a power propelling him towards the water, and he was able to walk upon the very waves. Thus he crossed the river.

When he heard the story, the master's joy knew no bounds. A swelling pride rose in his heart. Was it not his advice that had brought about the success? "I never knew that my advice had such great power," he thought. "Let me enjoy this miracle myself."

So he went to the river, which was now calm and serene, and uttered Krishna's name three times. Then he began to cross. But fear and doubt tortured his whole being, and although he shouted the sacred name hundreds of times, his attempt was fruitless. He drowned.

Now what do we learn from this story? The servant had sincere faith in his master. He also had an implicit faith in Lord Krishna. It was this absolute faith in a divine power that saved him and proved the power of Krishna's grace.

Similarly, a speaker, in spite of his own lame faith, can inspire a genuine faith in his listeners. But it is by being truly spiritual himself that he can help others most significantly. If we want to convince others of the Truth, our highest authority comes only from direct knowledge of Truth and not from any scripture. In the divine Play unillumined authority plays the role of the lamp, while Truth-in-realisation plays the role of the Light.

16.

Would you kindly advise me as to whether I should leave my wife and child in order to enter deeper into the spiritual life?

In your case, I feel that you should remain with your wife and child. Today you want to leave them; tomorrow you may want to leave God. It is not by leaving aside humanity that you will be able to realise God. If you remain with your family, your realisation will be deeper and more fulfilling. True, at a certain stage of the spiritual journey, the renunciation of the gross material life is necessary, but at a higher stage it is no longer necessary. At the highest stage, we neither seek nor renounce anything.

17.

Are spiritual experiences absolutely necessary to realise God?

No. There can be many roads leading to the same goal. One road may have many beautiful flowers on either side; another road may have only a few blossoms; a third road may have none at all. If three seekers each follow a different road according to their souls' needs and preferences, each of them will reach the Ultimate Goal.

Of course, experiences do give you additional confidence in yourself. They encourage you and energize you to march farther and farther. They also give enormous delight. And while you are having the experiences you may feel the presence of an invisible Guide within your being, pushing you towards the light of Truth so that you may be blessed with full Realisation.

But you can also have full and complete Realisation without so-called "experiences." Your expanding consciousness, as you grow into God, is itself a solid "experience."

18.

Why do you believe in rebirth? I know pretty well that I shall go to God when I die. And that's all.

My friend, as you will go to God when you leave the body, so will I. Let us be wise. Our business is to go to God; it is God's business if He wants to keep us in Heaven or send us back to earth. The best thing is to surrender to God and let Him fulfil us in His own way. Having thrown aside all our preconceived ideas regarding the existence or nonexistence of rebirth, let us do the only thing of importance: be one with His Will and Consciousness.

19.

Do you believe that in each incarnation the individual improves himself?

Yes, because he is evolving consciously or unconsciously.

20

Does the law of karma apply to everybody?

The law of *karma* applies to everyone, but one can transcend it through one's meditation. The law of *karma* exists and yet can be transcended by realisation, oneness with God and the power of spirituality.

21.

To pray to God or to work as God wants us to work: which is the better of the two?

I am happy to answer this question of questions. The answer is quite simple. To pray to God or to work as God wants us to work — both ways are of supreme importance. Both are certain means to an inevitable end. And that end is God-realisation.

22.

You said there are different ways of approaching God: action, devotion and knowledge. If one person possesses all these qualities, will it help his progress?

Certainly it helps. The attitude of service, the attitude of devotion and the quest for knowledge, taken all together, will help us make a balanced progress. But at some point in our life we will have to find the one that inspires us most and give it most importance. Each soul has its own way of moving. Here on earth, we are inspired to progress according to our soul's propensity. If we accept all these paths, it is a great help; at the same time, we have to pay most attention to our own soul's way, the way that gives us the greatest fulfilment according to our deepest aspiration.

23.

Will you please tell me something about meditation?

First you have to read a few spiritual books which explain the various ways to start meditation. Then you start. Soon you will see that reading books is not enough. You will feel that you need a teacher, who will know which kind of meditation will best suit your nature and soul. If you do not have a teacher, pray to God to reveal within you the kind of meditation you should adopt. Then, during a dream or in your silent mood, God will make you feel what you should do. Now you can begin your journey.

When your meditation is correct, you will feel a kind of joy all over your body. But if you do not feel that joy, if, on the contrary, you feel a mental tension or disturbance, then you should know that the kind of meditation you are doing is not meant for you and is not advisable. When you get a feeling of spontaneous inner joy, then the meditation you have adopted is correct.

24.

In order to come into closer contact with one's Self, to know the mysteries of one's inner Self, what is the correct procedure? I believe that meditation is where answers will be given about one's inner Self. Is this correct?

Yes, in meditation and concentration. Both will help. If you want to know your inner Self and learn about the inner mysteries of your life and the Universal Life, then you need meditation and concentration.

25.

Are there any set procedures one must follow in order to meditate correctly?

Each person has his own way of meditating. What actually happens is that sometimes an individual gets from within himself a kind of meditation. In other words, the inner being comes forward and tells the individual to pray or meditate in this or that way, that this or that will help. Sometimes the seeker meets a spiritual figure who can easily enter into him and know everything about his inner and outer life, seeing his growth and development and aspiration. Then this spiritual teacher can tell him how and when to meditate.

When you have a teacher you are extremely lucky, especially if the teacher is a genuine one.

If you don't have a teacher, but if you have genuine aspiration, God within you will tell you the correct meditation. It is not possible for everyone in the world to have a spiritual teacher. If you do not get one, what will happen? We are all God's children. God wants all of us to realise Him. So, if you get a teacher, well and good. If not, go deep within to discover your own meditation.

26.

But very often I may not recognize my inner Self. I do not know whether the voice I hear is the inner voice or the outer voice, and this is extremely confusing.

I fully understand. But if you get a teacher who is a realised soul, you can go to him for help and find out if what you are doing is correct. Or if you do not get a spiritual teacher, please go deep, deep within and see if you get a voice or a thought or an idea. Then go deep into the voice or thought or idea, and see if it gives you a feeling of inner joy or peace, where there are no questions or problems or doubts. When you get this kind of peace and inner joy, you can feel that the voice that you have heard is correct, that it is the real inner voice which will help you in your spiritual life.

27.

What is the difference between the voice of Silence and the voice of Yoga? Or isn't there any difference?

There is a difference. The voice of Silence will give you a particular piece of knowledge, a particular truth. When you enter into your inner being, into the inner realm where Silence really exists, if you need a particular message you will get it.

But Yoga encompasses everything; it is the whole field. In Yoga you will get Silence; you will also get Peace, Light and Power. You will get everything. The voice of Yoga is for all seekers and especially for those who have seriously entered into the spiritual life. The voice of Silence is meant for a particular seeker at a particular time. During your meditation, for example, you can go deep within and you will hear the voice of Silence. But the voice of Yoga you can have all the time. During your outer as well as your inner movements, you can hear the voice of Yoga. Since you have entered into the spiritual life, you will get spiritual vibrations, thoughts, ideas and messages. All these divine things will be coming to you from the voice of Yoga.

28.

When I try to meditate, I get a feeling of oceans and water before my mind's eye. This creates fear in me, and I cannot meditate very well. How can I meditate without getting this feeling of oceans and water?

Please try to see the ocean as something of your own, something in your inner being. Instead of seeing the ocean with its surges and waves, please think of it as your own largest consciousness, and throw yourself into that largest and deepest consciousness. Unfortunately, your attitude toward the ocean has been wrong. There are so many seekers who try to imagine the ocean during their meditation so that they can make their consciousness as vast as the ocean. When you see this consciousness, you should feel happy and fortunate.

Do not focus your attention on the surface of the ocean, but please go, silently and consciously, deep into the ocean, where you will find your true reality, which is all tranquility. Try to throw your own consciousness into the vastness of the ocean, and you will be able to meditate most powerfully and most successfully. You will be able to contact, deep within yourself, that which is nearest and dearest to your soul.

29

Sir, when did you come upon the thought that there is an inner Self within yourself? And after you discovered that you had an inner Self, how did you make a connection with other people who were not aware that they had an inner Self?

I have known intuitively, since my early childhood, that there is a deeper Self within me. Each one of us has an inner Self. Some are conscious of this inner Self and some are not. Those who are conscious of it are, according to us, spiritually developed. What they do in order to create a bridge between the outer world and the inner world, between the outer being and the inner being, is keep a burning flame of aspiration. This aspiration is based on self-sacrifice, outer and inner.

Suppose you have found your inner Self and inner life and discovered the solutions to your inner problems. But the person next door is utterly unconscious of the inner life and the inner world. Now it would be extremely difficult for you to have any kind of inner understanding with him. He cannot come and enter into your consciousness, for it is very difficult for an ordinary person to do this. But if you want to establish a bridge with him, what you can do during your meditation or concentration is this. First go deep within and bring forward all your sweet and subtle and harmonious feelings from within you. And then consciously, during your meditation, throw them into him: into his mind, into his body, into his heart. Then you have created a bridge between yourself and him.

Within your inner world you are secure. Your connection with the inner world has given you enormous confidence to cope with the outer world. Now you can go and speak to him about the spiritual life, the inner life, the life that gives you true happiness. He can then try it for himself.

So first within yourself, just like watering a plant every day, feed your inner being by meditation. Then come to the outer world with your creative manifestation to form a bridge between your inner achievements and the outer world, where your future fulfilment will take place.

30.

There are seven planes of consciousness in the spiritual development. How can I determine which plane I belong to?

You can know which plane you belong to by throwing your outer mind into the sea of your aspiring heart, whose source is Consciousness. This Consciousness is the life-breath of all planes. The awareness of this Consciousness permits you immediately to recognize your status — where you were, where you are now and how far you still have to go.

After becoming aware of which plane you belong to, try to carry out all your daily activities on that level. The easiest and most effective way of operating from that plane is to make your outer being a conscious and dedicated instrument of your inner vision and will.

In your case, let us suppose that you want to act from the intuitive mind. Once you have seen that plane and are conscious of it, you can try to remain there through your psychic aspiration and determined will. This is the real way to achieve mastery over a particular plane.

31.

You are always using the word "conscious-ness." What exactly does it mean?

I will give you a very simple definition. Consciousness is the spark of life which connects each one of us with the Universal Life. It is the thread that puts us in tune with the universe. If you want to fly into the Transcendental, you need the thread of consciousness.

Consciousness is a spark that lets us enter into the Light. It is our consciousness which connects us with God. It is the link between God and man, between Heaven and earth.

32.

Do we have control of our consciousness?

An ordinary man does not have control of his

consciousness. But a spiritual man is able to control his. He tries to lead a better life, a higher life, and in so doing, he brings down the Light of the Beyond into the darkness of the present-day world.

33.

How do I work on my consciousness?

Don't think of doing anything. Just keep the door of your consciousness open, but see whether it is a thief or a friend who is coming in. Allow in only those whom you want. Keep out the lower thoughts. Open the door to higher, sublime thoughts. This is the first step in working on your consciousness. The following steps will come to you from within.

34.

What is the meaning of AUM?

AUM is a Sanskrit word, a syllable. A Sanskrit word or a syllable has a special significance and a creative power. AUM is the Mother of all sounds. When we chant AUM, what actually happens is that we bring down Peace and Light from above and create a universal harmony within us and without us. When we repeat AUM, both our inner and our outer being become inspired and surcharged with a divine feeling and aspiration. AUM has no equal. AUM has infinite power. Just by repeating AUM, we can realise God.

When you chant AUM, try to feel that it is God who is climbing up and down within you. Hundreds of seekers in India have realised God simply by repeating AUM. AUM is the symbol of God, the Creator.

When you repeat AUM, please try to observe what actually happens. If you repeat the name of a cat, a dog or a monkey, or even of an ordinary person, you get no inspiration. But when you utter AUM, which is the symbol of the Creator, the life-breath of the Creator, you immediately get an inner feeling, a feeling that inspires your inner and outer movements to enlarge your vision and fulfil your life here on earth. This is the secret of AUM. If you want to cherish a secret all your life, then here is the secret. Soulfully chant AUM and everything is yours.

35.

Is it better to meditate on AUM or on God?

Everything has its own time. I have just told you about the significance of AUM, and the other day I told you about God. You have to know in which word you have more faith. When one person says God, all his love, faith and devotion come to the fore. In someone else, this may not be so. In your case, I told you to repeat the name of God, for you go to church and pray in the Christian way. In your culture, you are familiar with the term God.

In India, we repeat AUM or the name of a god or goddess, such as Shiva, Krishna or Kali. The most important thing is to know in whom or in which aspect of the Supreme you have absolute faith. When I told you about God, I had the feeling that all your life you had been trained to pray to God. But today AUM enters into you with its significance. One day I shall meditate with you and see whether God, AUM, Supreme, Infinite or some other aspect of the Absolute inspires you most. It is the inspiration that you get which is of the utmost importance.

36.

Is God a mental being?

We have a physical body and a mind. Similarly, we can think of God as a physical being, having a mind like ours. People often imagine God as composed of a gigantic mind, or else functioning like them with the mind. Up until now, the mind has been humanity's greatest achievement. With the help of the mind, science and our physical world have progressed to an enormous extent. As the mind has been our highest attainment, we tend to think of God as a being with a most highly developed mind. But God is not a mental being. God does not act from the mind. He does not need the mental formulations which we utilize in order to act.

God does not need to formulate ideas in a mental way.

Human beings usually think before they act. But in God's case, it is not like that. He uses His Willpower which, while seeing, also acts and becomes. God's seeing, acting and becoming are simultaneous and instantaneous.

37.

How can one move ultimately toward success, believing that "As thy feet bend, so bends the path"? Is that really possible?

It is quite possible. We think we must have a plan first so we can achieve success in the future by progressing and achieving according to our plan. Now we are labouring with our minds. The mind says, "I have to achieve something. I have to think about how I can execute my plan." But God does not do that. God sees the past, present and future at a glance. When we are one with God, when — by constant aspiration — we identify ourselves with God's Consciousness, then whatever we do will be done spontaneously. Then we will not utilize the mind, but always act from our own inner consciousness, with our intuitive faculty. And when we develop that intuitive faculty, we can easily act without having a plan.

At each moment, the possibility of the total manifestation that is going to take place will materialize right in front of us. Now we think that within, let us say, ten or twenty days some possibility may materialize concerning our hopes and aspirations. But when we are one with God's Consciousness, it is more than a possibility. It is an inevitability, an immediate achievement. The vision and the fulfilment go together. In the ordinary human consciousness, the vision is one thing and the fulfilment is something else. But when we are one with God's Consciousness, the vision and the fulfilment are inseparable.

38.

About the vision and its fulfilment, how do you know that you are having the right "vision"?

Are you referring to yourself or are you speaking generally? If it is yourself, I can tell you easily. I know that in your meditation there are times when you go very deep, and your inner voice tells you, on the spur of the moment, that something has already been done. Your mind does not come and impose its ideas on that voice, saying, "If you do this, perhaps it will be a mistake; don't do that, or something may happen in the future; if you do it . . . and if you don't do it . . ." etc. The mind does not interfere. You can rest assured that when you get this kind of vision in your deep meditation, it is correct and it will spontaneously bring its own fulfilment.

39

Guru Chinmoy, you were speaking about the vision without the mind. Is this what is known as intuition? Or is intuition something else?

You may call it either intuition or the direct perception of Truth, which needs no mental help. It is knowledge without thought or mental form. It is direct and spontaneous. It makes you feel what it is. Normally, you see something and then you give it a mental form, saying "This is what it is." But intuition simply makes you feel its true existence at once. Intuition houses the depth of Vision and the wealth of Realisation all together.

40.

Is the mind itself a kind of machine connecting the higher and the lower?

The mind is a link. Through the mind you can go to the regions far above the mind. But at the same time, through the mind, you can come to your vital being, your lower vital being. The mind is a channel that links us with what is above and what is below.

41.

In the old books they talk about Nama-Rupa, *Name and Form. Words are* Nama-Rupa, *right?*

Ideas are Nama-Rupa. *Now this is not really God. These are human concoctions. The meaning is a manufactured thing. There is no reality in the word itself, true?*

As you know, the study of semantics has gone into this problem very deeply. We know that it is not the actual word but the concept which we attach to the word that creates most of our difficulties. It is not the word itself that has an intrinsic value, but what concept the word conveys to us. But certain spiritual words are surcharged with a meaning or a condition or a consciousness that has developed in them from thousands of years of a special spiritual usage. When we enter deeply into the significance of such a word, and reveal its very breath and manifest its inner reality on the outer level, then the word fulfils its purpose, both inwardly and outwardly.

The spiritual approach to the problem of words is that we have to go from the form to the Formless. We have to go through the finite to the Infinite. Indeed, this is the divine logic. Form at the beginning has a peerless value, but not necessarily at the end. For the beginner on the spiritual path, a form is absolutely necessary; the form is everything to him. So in the beginning we say that God has a form. But when the seeker goes deep within and sees that God is not a human being or a mental being but a vast infinite Consciousness, he goes beyond the form to the Formless, and can feel God as the infinite

Consciousness. But again, God, being Infinite, can also be finite. Otherwise, He would not be Infinite. He is Omnipotent because He can live in the tiny atom and in the vast universe at the same time.

42.

Sri Chinmoy, in the Hindu tradition one speaks of how Atman *equals* Brahman — *the individual soul equals the Universal Soul. Jesus Christ once said, "I and my Father are one." These two statements, coming from two different spiritual backgrounds — are they, in the spiritual light, one and the same?*

It is the same statement. *Atman* and *Paramatman* are the individual soul and the Supreme Self. God comes down into the manifestation and takes the form of the individual soul, *Atman.* Then the individual soul in the process of its evolution reaches and becomes the Supreme Self, *Paramatman.* To fulfil Himself integrally and wholly in the material world, God needs the individual soul.

The statements are the same. When Christ said, "I and my Father are one," it was like saying that *Atman* and *Paramatman* are one. That is why in India we say *Atmanam Viddhi,* "Know Thyself." If you know yourself, then you know God, because in essence there is no difference between you and God. Self-realisation is God-realisation and God-realisation is Self-realisation. For this reason in India we also say *Soham asmi,* "He am I," and *Aham Brahma,* "I am Brahman." In the same vein, all the esoteric traditions have always maintained that true knowledge is found by seeking within. This is why Jesus said, "The Kingdom of Heaven is within you."

43.

Would you care to elaborate on the statement, "The Kingdom of Heaven is within you"?

First let me say that it is science that has greatly contributed to the general feeling that Heaven is a place outside of ourselves. Science has exercised its power on the conscious and sub-conscious planes of human thinking. The twentieth-century idea of Heaven, in the West at any rate, is leading mankind in the wrong direction in its conception of Heaven.

The Kingdom of Heaven is something that we can feel, and not something that we can demonstrate. Science can demonstrate many things. But the Kingdom of Heaven is a matter of our own inner achievement. If we have realised the Kingdom of Heaven within ourselves, others will look at us and feel that we have something quite unusual, unearthly and supernal. Because we have seen and felt and possessed the Kingdom of Heaven within ourselves, they will regard us as a totally transformed extraordinary being.

Needless to say, it is our aspiration, our

mounting inner cry, that leads us to this Kingdom of Heaven. The Kingdom of Heaven is a plane full of Peace and Delight. We feel it when we reside deep within ourselves and when we transcend our egocentric individual consciousness. The higher we go beyond our limited consciousness, the quicker we enter into our deepest, infinite consciousness, the more intimately we shall see, feel and possess the Kingdom of Heaven within ourselves.

To be sure, the Kingdom of Heaven is more than just a mere plane, like other planes. It is a plane of divine Consciousness. It is a state of Realisation. It embodies *Sat-Chit-Ananda*. *Sat* is divine Existence, *Chit* is divine Consciousness, *Ananda* is divine Bliss. When we go deep within, we feel these three together, and when we acquire the inner vision to perceive them all at once, we live verily in the Kingdom of Heaven. Otherwise, Existence is at one place, Consciousness is somewhere else and Bliss is nowhere near the other two. When we see and feel Existence-Consciousness-Bliss on the selfsame plane, each complementing and fulfilling the others, we can say that we live in the Kingdom of Heaven. Yes, the Kingdom of Heaven is within us. Not only can we feel it, but without the least possible doubt, we can become it.

44.

What exactly is the ego?

The ego is that very thing which limits us in every sphere of life. We are God's children; we are one with God. But the ego makes us feel that we do not belong to God, that we are perfect strangers to Him. At best, it makes us feel that we are going to God, not that we are *in* God.

The ordinary human ego gives us a sense of separate identity, separate consciousness. No doubt, a sense of individuality and self-importance is necessary at a certain stage in man's development. But the ego separates our individual consciousness from the Universal Consciousness. The very function of the ego is separation. It cannot feel satisfaction in viewing two things at a time on the same level. It always feels that one must be superior to the other. So the ego makes us feel that we are all separate weaklings, that it will never be possible for us to be or to have the Infinite Consciousness. The ego, finally, is limitation. This limitation is ignorance, and ignorance is death. So ego ultimately ends in death.

45.

How was the ego born? How did it come into being?

The ego came into existence from limitation. The moment the soul enters into the physical consciousness or the physical world, it is in a strange, foreign world. In spite of being a flame of the Divine and, in essence, omnipotent, the soul in the beginning finds it very difficult to cope with the world. And even later, when the person grows older, most of the time the soul has to endure unpleasant experiences just in order to remain in the physical world and, more importantly, to establish the Divine here on earth.

The ego each day gets the opportunity to function independently and gets stronger day by day, until it separates itself completely from the source of its absolute, divine fulfilment: the soul. The ego, which wants to starve and crush the Divine in man, is fed by the ignorance of the physical world. The Divine, too, initially feeds the ego, but later illumines and transforms it into a perfect instrument of the Supreme.

46.

How do we weaken the ego and ultimately subdue it?

By thinking of God's all-pervading Consciousness. This Consciousness is not something that we have to achieve. This Consciousness is already within us; we have just to be aware of it. Further, while we are in meditation we have to develop it and illumine it to infinite proportions. And to our wide surprise, the ego will be buried in the bosom of death.

THE FOLLOWING QUESTIONS WERE ASKED BY CHILDREN

47.

Gurudev, I want to ask you something. If I break an egg, can God put it together again?

Certainly He can. God can do anything He wants.

48.

Can you do it?

No. Sorry, Shannon, your Gurudev cannot do it. But if God gives me the power, I can easily do it.

49.

Can I do it?

Why not? The moment God gives you the power, you can easily put a broken egg together again. A day will come when you, I and everyone will have the same power that God has now.

50.

Is it true that anybody can become a yogi if he really tries?

What do you mean by *really*? If you mean sincerely, then certainly anybody can become a yogi.

Yoga means union with God. A yogi is he who is one with God. Sooner or later, all human beings will realise God. But the person who takes to Yoga reaches God sooner. If you yourself want to become a yogini and realise God, then right now start praying. Especially if you want to reach God before the rest of humanity, please do not delay.

Now, how do you go about praying? If you pray to God for candy today, tomorrow you will ask Him for ice cream and the day after tomorrow for something else. And God will give you everything that you want, except Himself. But if you pray to God only for Himself and nothing else, He will give you all that He has and all that He is. In getting all that He has and all that He is, not only will you get your candy and ice cream and everything else that you wanted, but you will also get things that you had never imagined, things of an infinite nature. So pray to God every day to give you what you need and not what you want. Then He will give you what you actually need to become one with Him.

51.

What does God look like?

When I look at you, God looks exactly as you do. If I look at your mother, God looks like your mother. And if I look at someone else, then God looks like him. If I should look within myself, I would find that God looks like Chinmoy. Although you may not see this now, when you are able to see deep within yourself, you will know that each of us cannot be considered separately from God.

Now I am holding my two fingers together. As you see, if I try I can pull them apart. But if, rather than fingers, they were you and God, I could not separate them, no matter how hard I tried. In fact, the more I tried to separate the two of you, the tighter you would stick together.

Because God is in you, God looks exactly like you. Right now, you are God veiled. You have put on a mask, but I see through the mask. In the future, you will be the God unveiled. You will take off the mask and we shall see you as God manifested, the open God.

52.

How come you can see God and I can't?

This is such a nice question. Now you are looking at me with your eyes open. You are looking at me, Chinmoy, and you are able to see me. Now *(putting his hands over her eyes)*, I have closed your eyes. Can you see me? No, you cannot see me. When your eyes are shut you cannot see anybody. But when you keep your eyes open, you can see me, you can see your father, your friends, everyone.

Now you have another eye which is between your eyebrows, and just slightly above. It is your inner eye, your Third Eye. In my case that eye is open. I have kept it open. So I can see God, and I can see everything that is within others. Now Shannon, in your case, just as you cannot see anything when your two eyes are closed, so also you do not see God because your Third Eye is closed.

If you pray to God every day, someday this inner eye will open up. Get up early in the morning and open your two ordinary eyes and see your mother and father and everything that is in your room and then pray to God. One day, as a result of your prayer, you will see that your Third Eye has opened, and you also will be able to see God, just as you see me now.

God is close to us because He is
*   the Supreme Lover.*
We are far from Him because we are
*   eternal doubters.*

QUESTIONS AND ANSWERS ON THE SOUL

1.

Is the soul always with the person during his lifetime, or can it leave him temporarily, even making its home elsewhere?

As a rule, the soul always remains with the person during his lifetime, but it can leave the body for a few minutes, or a few hours at most, while the person is asleep. It can also leave the body for a short period while the aspirant is in a deep state of meditation. Then one can see one's own body. One may see it as a dead body or a dynamic body or as a shaft of light facing his soul, or in many other ways. Of course, at that time, one sees the body with the eye of his own soul.

2.

During sleep, does the person's soul make journeys?

Yes. The soul makes journeys to different

levels of consciousness. There are seven higher worlds and seven lower worlds. Generally the soul travels in these worlds during sleep. Almost everyone's soul is fortunate enough to have access to some of these worlds, but very few are conscious of these experiences while they are happening, or remember them after they awake.

3.

Can a person's body and consciousness so change during his lifetime that he becomes fit for a finer soul to enter him?

A finer soul does not enter him. But if the person's body and consciousness are transformed totally, then the soul that he already possesses will be in a position to fulfil its divine mission here on earth most effectively, in all its supernal Perfection.

4.

Does a change, such as purification, during the lifetime, change the soul?

It is the same soul. Previously it accepted ignorance, but now, throwing away the veil of ignorance, it comes closer to its own divine plenitude and divine manifestation.

5.

When we think another's thoughts, we let ourselves tune in to his "psychic" agitations. However, if we tune in to one whom we believe to be grounded in the Source of his being, his soul, would this be a valid practice, at least until our own spiritual unfolding developed?

First of all, let us be clear about the use of the word "psychic." As I use it, "psychic" is not a synonym for "occult," but pertains to the psychic being. There is no agitation in the psychic being, which is a divine spark, to say the least. We usually let ourselves tune in to others' vital or mental agitations. Certainly it is a valid practice to tune in to an enlightened soul. That is what one should do in the beginning or until one has the capacity to unfold oneself spiritually. That is why we say that if you remain calm and quiet and allow the divine thoughts of your spiritual Guide to enter into you, you will become flooded with Peace. This kind of tuning in is not only a valid and correct practice, but is essential for one who has placed himself under the guidance of a spiritual Master.

6.

How does one know if his soul is happy?

First of all, one has to know and feel where the soul abides, its location in the body. In order to know and feel the soul, one has to aspire. During one's ardent aspiration, one's spiritual journey, one can actually discover whether the soul is happy or not. He will feel that his soul is happy only when he sees and feels joy within and without, and also when he does not find fault with God's creation and God's divine dispensation.

7.

Does the soul cry when it is unhappy?

No. The real soul, which is a portion of the Cosmic Self, is all Delight. Since it cannot be unhappy in the human sense of the term, it does not cry. It is the unsatisfied and demanding vital, which we often take for the soul, that suffers unhappiness and cries pitifully.

8.

Are there two sets of instructions within the person, one from his deepest nature — which includes and unfolds all in goodness and compassion — and the other, which is clever about "me" and "mine"?

Yes. There are two sets of instructions within the person. Goodness and compassion come from the very depth of one's being, whereas "me" and "mine" come from the surface. "Me" and "mine" cannot come from the very depths.

9.

Can the soul be equally represented in dreams by an old woman, wrinkled and wise, as well as by a young baby babbling a new language?

Yes. The soul can be represented in dreams by an old woman or by a young baby. In order to give a particular experience to the outer being, the soul can assume any form in dreams. The gradual divine maturity of the soul can be compared to the gradual growth of a seed into a tree.

10.

Is the soul both male and female?

The soul itself is neither male nor female. But when the soul at the start of its human journey takes a female body, then in all its future incarnations it will take a female body. If it first takes a male body, then in all its incarnations it will take a male body. It is nearly impossible to change the sex. In the whole history of mankind there have been a few exceptions here and there, but very rarely.

11.

Is it the soul that makes the decision in selecting a new body in each incarnation?

Yes. It is the soul that makes the decision in

selecting a body, but with the direct approval of the Supreme or the Self. The choice is made to give the soul the opportunity to manifest more and more of its inner divinity in each incarnation and to fulfil the Will of the Divine here on earth.

12.

Is it the soul that must surrender to the Cosmic Self?

Yes. Each human being has an individual soul. This soul has to surrender to the Self — the Self which, in Indian terms, is called *Paramatman,* and is unmanifest. This Self does not take human incarnation or enter into creation, whereas the soul takes a human body and accepts limitation, imperfection and ignorance. This individual soul, which takes a human body, is not all-pervading, omniscient or omnipotent. The Self is. The soul, in its upward evolution, can some day merge into the Self and become as powerful as the Self.

13.

Does the soul get new instruction in its development, or does it merely uncover what it has always known?

If you say "experience" rather than "instruction," the question would be more accurate. Only God, or the Cosmic Self, can instruct the soul.

116

The soul is uncovering what it has always known. But at the same time, it is growing and enriching itself by taking into itself the divine essence of its earthly experiences. Meanwhile, the physical consciousness is becoming more and more conscious of the soul's unlimited divine capacity. In essence, the soul, being one with God, is uncovering what it has always known. But in the process of evolution, its *becoming* and *knowing, knowing* and *becoming* move together and are complementary processes in the lap of the Supreme Truth.

14.

Does the soul experience loneliness? If so, how does this differ from our superficial need to have the company of others, regardless of whether we like them or not, simply because we want someone to talk to?

The soul experiences loneliness only when the body, vital, mind and heart, which are supposed to co-operate with the soul in fulfilling its divine mission on earth, do not co-operate. At that time it experiences loneliness. But it does not act like a human being. It does not waste its time, like a human being who feels that if he just talks to others his sense of loneliness will disappear. The soul, in its loneliness, aspires most intensely to bring down Peace, Light and Power from above into the physical, the vital and the mental so that the total being can co-operate with the soul to fulfil the Divine. When Peace, Light and Power descend this way, the person becomes conscious of his inner life and true happiness. With Peace, Light and Power a higher consciousness descends. With this higher consciousness, the person will naturally respond to the soul's need.

15.

Does the soul make demands on a person so that he has to change his ways?

The soul does not make demands as such. It is not like a mother making demands of her child at every moment, saying, "I'm telling you such and such for your own good." What the soul does is send a divine inspiration. This inspiration can at times be so vivid and spontaneous that the person may feel it to be almost an inner imposition made by his inner self on his outer personality. But the soul does not demand. On the contrary, it sympathizes with human failings and imperfections and tries to identify itself with these failings. And then, with its inner Light, it tries to help the person to change his ways.

16.

How different is this from the demands the ego makes?

We now know that the soul does not make any demands. When the ego makes a demand, it is all self-centred — "I," "me," "mine." The ego wants to possess and be possessed. By feeding the outer personality, the ego wants to fulfil itself. But this is simply impossible, as there is no end to its cravings. When the soul wants to have something, it is not for its own personal benefit but for the fulfilment of the Divine. The ego eventually meets with frustration, whereas the soul, by fulfilling the Divine Will, realises its own absolute fulfilment.

17.

When the vital or mental tries to satisfy itself without the soul's approval, what happens to the soul?

In such cases the soul usually remains silent. But at times the Supreme may put some pressure on the vital and the mind when they are going too far. He does this through the soul.

18.

Do things or places have a soul? For example, does a chair have a soul, does a city have a soul?

Each thing and each place has a soul. Like all other cities, the city of New York has a soul. The Supreme has graciously shown me the soul of New York City a number of times. The difference between the souls of things and the souls of humans is a matter of their degree of evolution, the degree to which they manifest their divine potentialities. It is through the process of reincarnation that the soul gradually manifests its hidden powers within, and eventually reaches its absolute Fulfilment.

19.

Does the earth have a soul?

Certainly. The earth represents the Mother aspect of the Divine. It is on earth that Matter and Spirit will find their absolute fulfilment through their reciprocal help and complete union. Matter will see through the eye of the Spirit's vision. Spirit will flower by awakening and energizing Matter to become a perfect basis of physical immortality and human transformation on earth. The two main characteristics of the soul of the earth are aspiration and compassionate tolerance.

20.

Can the gross ever give the subtle anything? That is, can the soul become stronger by the right use of the body such as exercise, right food, and so on?

Certainly. The gross can and must help the subtle. The body is gross, but in its sound and perfect condition, it helps the mind and the subtle existence considerably. One cannot, of course, make the soul stronger merely by taking vigorous physical exercises or by eating judiciously. But if the body, that is, the physical consciousness, aspires to grow in the Light of the soul and tries to fulfil the Divine in the physical itself, then the progress of the soul becomes easier, faster and more fulfilling.

21.

Can the soul select what the individual is to experience in the manifested world?

Normally it is the soul that determines the experiences that the individual will have in his lifetime. As a matter of fact, if the individual consciously puts himself into the spontaneous flow of experiences that the soul wants to give him, he will eventually grow into abiding peace, joy and fulfilment. Unfortunately, the individual, being a victim of ignorance, is often not aware of the experiences the soul selects, or in spite of knowing, does not care for the selection made by the soul.

22.

Approximately where in the physical body does one feel a sense of soul?

It is in the spiritual heart. According to medical science, the heart is slightly to the left of the centre of the chest. According to Ramana Maharshi, the great sage of Arunachala, the spiritual heart is slightly to the right of centre. Some spiritual figures say that the heart is in the middle of the chest. But, according to one spiritual figure, the spiritual heart is located between the eyebrows! Of course, he also has his reasons for saying this.

The true spiritual heart, about four finger-breadths in width, is located approximately twelve finger-breadths directly above the navel and six finger-breadths directly below the centre of the throat. It is here that one feels what you have called the "quickening" of the soul.

23.

If the body or personality is the newcomer and the soul is the real landlord, or lord, then how is it that the newcomer, which is always seeking satisfaction, can so suffocate the soul that its inspiration cannot be heard?

I am happy to answer this particular question. The *Katha Upanishad* says that the body is the chariot, the mind is the reins, the intellect is the charioteer and the soul is the master of the chariot.

You are the landlady of the building in which we have our Centre. You own this building. We are your tenants. We are all newcomers. You try your best to satisfy our requirements. Nevertheless, not all, but some of the tenants make your life a hell. Their demands are at times outrageous and absurd. Further, they cherish an uncompromising attitude. What do you do then? I believe you become quite helpless, if not hopeless, in spite of the fact that it is you who own this building. It is not easy to drive away the disturbing, demanding, uncompromising tenants all at once. Similar is the fate of the soul which is attacked by the pleasure-seeking, demanding and unaspiring newcomer, the personality.

24.

When someone is described as having a young soul or an old soul, what does this mean?

From the spiritual point of view, when one has acquired higher and deeper experiences from previous incarnations, one is called an old soul. The person who is wanting in such experiences is called a young soul. As you can see, it is not the number of incarnations that determines the "status" of the soul, but what one has learned and achieved in those lives.

25.

Do things move faster with a young soul because there is less overlay from previous incarnations?

Things do move faster with a young soul provided that he is a sincere and dedicated aspirant, that he listens to his spiritual Guide unreservedly and that he has not been burdened with too many worldly experiences.

Here again we have to be aware of one thing: it is not the number of incarnations that impedes the soul's rapid journey toward its Ultimate Goal, but the old unlit human habits and propensities which do not open so easily to the Light for purification and transformation.

26.

What is the difference between "strength of soul" and "strength of character"?

Strength of character is the pride of morality and humanity. Strength of soul is the pride of Spirituality, Eternity and Infinity. Having said this, I do not want to leave you with the impression that morality has no value in the inner and spiritual life. On the contrary, a solid morality is preparatory to a deep spirituality. Strength of soul is the inner power or certitude that comes from the Divine within you. When you have seen your soul, you have felt God's Will within you and you have been given the strength to manifest His Will here on earth.

27.

Could the soul that inhabits a human body have inhabited an animal body or a plant in previous times?

I am sure you are well acquainted with the theory of evolution. Charles Darwin, in the modern world, discovered the process of the evolution of species, that is, the change from a lower form to a higher form. But long before Darwin, a thousand years before the advent of the Christ, the great Indian sage, Kapila, had discovered the theory of spiritual evolution. The Eternal, Unchangeable and Imperishable at every moment evolves: this was his unique philosophy. Nothing came from nothing. The Indian sage discovered this truth and offered it to the world at large.

The total process of evolution on earth includes the soul as well as the physical form. In the march of evolution, each soul has to go through the plant life and the animal life before it can launch into the human life.

28.

Do souls differ in their characteristics?

There is actually no basic difference among souls except in the degree of their manifestation. All souls possess the same possibilities, whether they are housed in the lowest or the highest form of life.

We have to remember, however, that the Supreme manifests Himself in infinite ways through the different souls. They express His varying aspects of Divinity. For example, one soul may manifest Light, another Power, a third

Beauty, and so on.

It is by manifesting their hidden potentialities through the process of reincarnation that some souls have become great spiritual Masters. And all souls shall eventually follow them.

29.

What is the connection of the soul to past and future karma?

Actually, *karma* cannot be truly understood apart from the soul. It is for the sake of the soul's growth that *karma* exists. You know, I am sure, what the word *karma* means. It is a Sanskrit word, derived from the root *kri,* "to do." Whatever we do, say or think is *karma.* The universe is governed by a law which we call the Law of *Karma.* You have read much about the Law of *Karma,* so I need not explain it here, except to say that all one's deeds and thoughts leave their impression upon one's causal body and bring about certain results.

At the same time, the soul is far beyond the snare of cause and effect. It is the hyphen between all that precedes and all that succeeds. It is enriched by all the experiences which the personality derives through the laws of *karma.*

30

Where does the soul rest when it first leaves the body? Does it carry over its bodily or earthly limitations?

When the soul leaves the body, it first stays in the vital world for a short period. Some souls suffer there; others do not. It is like visiting a strange, new country. Some are fortunate enough to mix freely with the people of the new country and understand its culture in almost no time, while others are not so fortunate.

The soul does not carry over any earthly limitations to the higher worlds. The soul or psychic being, while leaving the body and going back to its own region, gathers together the quintessence of its earthly experiences. It stays for some time in its own region and then it comes back into this world with a new determination and new possibilities to realise and fulfil the Divine here on earth.

I and My Beloved

I am my Beloved's. Lo, His spontaneous Love flows toward me. My Beloved is mine. Lo, my spontaneous cry carries me toward Him.

PART THREE:

RELIGION (MAINLY HINDUISM)

Surrender

O loving surrender, God wants you.
O devoted surrender, God needs you.
O all-giving surrender, God embraces you
and cherishes you.

WHAT IS RELIGION?

What is religion? Religion is God. Religion is Truth. God and Truth are one. But when I say that my religion is God, there is every possibility that you may misunderstand me. But if I say that my religion is Truth, immediately you see eye to eye with me. Let me be a little clearer. If I say that my religion is Lord Krishna and you must accept him, your eyes emit fire. But if I say that my religion is Truth, you will jump up and say, "So is mine." Now, instead of saying, "You must accept my religion," if I say, "Let us accept the universal Truth," you will cry out, "Already accepted, thank you, my friend!"

Religion is an act of vision that guides and leads us to the Beyond. Religion is intuition. Intuition is so near and dear to each of us, so familiar to our soul and so intimate to our heart, that it requires no definition. Even so, we may as well proclaim the truth that intuition is the consciousness of the all-pervading existence. Ask a man how he is sure of his existence. Silence captures his mouth. He knows what his existence is. He feels it. But the explanation evades him. Religion is that very intuition which defies explanation but which is a self-embodying and self-explanatory truth.

Religion is not fanaticism. Religion, in its purest form, is a feeling of the universal oneness of Truth. A fanatic never sees the truth in its totality, even in his wildest imagination. A fanatic has nothing to offer to the world precisely because he has not kept his heart's door wide open, and because he lacks the capacity to commune with his soul.

What we need is direct Illumination. Lo, differences are buried in oblivion. Through our feeling of universal oneness, we run closer and closer to the Supreme. Our life has a freedom of its own. Our narrowness in thought kills this freedom. This freedom finds no joy in lofty and grandiose pronouncements. This freedom wants to be the living expression of our inner thoughts and feelings. Freedom is union. Union is the all-energizing and all-fulfilling Truth.

Religion speaks. It speaks more significantly than words. Unfortunately, its message is often subject to our ruthless distortion. Nevertheless, in the long run, it triumphantly voices forth the truth.

When we think of religion, our attitude should be sympathetic and appreciative rather than critical and competitive. Criticism and competition create disharmony, which is a destructive force. Sympathy and appreciation create harmony, which is a creative force. Harmony, moreover, is the life of existence.

All religions are indispensable to their adherents. All religions, too, are surcharged with inspiration. This inspiration is the conviction of the adherents' collective soul. Peace must be their watchword, just as Truth is their sole aim.

Momentous are the words of Tagore, who said of religion:

> "Religion, like poetry, is not a mere idea; it is expression. The self-expression of God is in the endless variedness of creation; and our attitude towards the Infinite Being must also in its expression have a variedness of individuality, ceaseless and unending."

Religion is a living challenge to the highest in human beings to face the stormy problems of life. True, there are countless problems. But there is also an Omnipotent Power. Strangely enough, this power utilizes the problems as true instruments for the future blessing of humanity.

Religion expands. It expands our feelings. Religion lives. It lives in the inmost recesses of our heart. Religion conquers. It conquers in our self-giving.

The divine aim of religion is to release the pent-up reservoir of human energy. Life itself is religion — intimate, continuous and fulfilling. Let us live openly and freely. Let us have that religion which includes all human beings who have ever lived on earth, those who are now on the world stage and those who shall dwell here during untold ages to come. Ours is the religion that will perfect the order of the world. Ours is the religion that will ply between the shores of Eternity and Infinity.

THE UNIVERSALITY OF RELIGION

The Universalist Church of New York is for all religions of the world. It is a growing family with one Home. This Home is the embodiment of Heart. Heart is the embodiment of Truth. Fulfilment is there where Truth is.

Why do we need religion? We need religion because we want to go beyond the finite in order to commune with the Infinite. This is not only possible but also inevitable, for in us there is a conscious being which envisions God's Reality in totality.

Religion is a spontaneous experience and never a theoretical knowledge. This experience is immensely practical, and we can use it consciously at every moment of our earthly existence.

Religion has never been thrust upon man. It has sprung from the deepest need of his inner being. When this inner being comes to the fore and looks around, it feels God's all-permeating Immanence; and when it looks up, it feels God's all-surpassing Transcendence as its own divine heritage.

Religion has two lives: the outer and the inner. It offers its outer life to seekers in the preliminary stage of vital and emotional aspiration. It offers its inner life to the universal meditation and God-realisation.

Religion in the physical is an unconscious cry for God; in the vital, a blind struggle to possess God; in the mind, a constant fight to conquer God; in the heart, a conscious cry to sit in the Lap of God; and in the soul, a Consciousness-boat that longs to ply between the shores of the ever-transcending Infinity and the ever-blooming Immortality.

Immorality wants to blight religion. God says to religion: "Fear not, My child, I am giving you the indomitable strength of morality." Egoism wants to suffocate religion. God says to religion: "Fear not, My child, I am placing you in the ever-widening vastness of universality." Death wants to devour religion. God says to religion: "Fear not, My child, I am making you the embodiment of immortality."

Science and religion. People say that science and religion are always at daggers drawn. This need not be true. Science plays its role dynamically in explaining the immanent God. Religion plays its role divinely in interpreting the transcendent God. Science deals with the physical world, while religion deals with the inner and spiritual world. Mind is the student and Nature is the professor of science. Heart is the student and Soul is the professor of religion.

Philosophy and religion. Philosophy and religion are two intimate friends. Philosophy reaches its acme of perfection when it is inspired by the faith, vision, experience and realisation of soulful religion. And with the help of alert and sound philosophy, religion frees itself from the snares of superstition, vagary and fantasy.

Morality and spirituality in religion. Morality in religion is a steady journey toward an ideal life. This journey at times appears to be a never-ending one. Nevertheless, it embodies an approximation of the ideal visualized, the goal. Spirituality in religion is fully aware of its implicit Infinity. It transports an aspiring individual into the living Abode of God. The Infinity that spirituality reveals in religion is actualized through a spontaneous inner urge. For the religious aspirant, hope flies into certainty, struggle enters into conquest and willpower is beckoned by absolute Fulfilment.

Individuality and universality. Universality does not and cannot mean an utter extinction of the mounting individual flame in the human heart. On the contrary, when the individual transcends himself in the continuous process of universalization, he will most assuredly abide in the deeper, vaster and higher realms of Light, Peace and Power. Only then will he grow into his own true Self, his Self Eternal. No doubt, at the very beginning, he will feel a deplorable conflict between individuality and universality. But this feeling of his will not last forever, for the self-same conflict contains within itself the possibility of a most convincing concord, a pure amalgam of unique transcendence.

Religious faith. Religion without faith is a body without life in it. Religious faith is a transforming experience and not just an idea. Faith has the magic key to self-discovery. Self-discovery is the bona fide discovery of Reality. Faith is an active participant in divine Love, Harmony and Peace. Finally, it transports religion into the all-pervading Delight of the Beyond.

Sin in religion. It is true that the conception of sin looms large in religion. What is sin? It is nothing but an experience of imperfection. This imperfection exists simply because creation is still in the making. Perfection must needs dawn on creation. It is a matter of time. Creation is action, a constant movement: forward, upward and inward. Evolution is the immortal song which is perpetually sung by creation. Today's sin is imperfection personified. Tomorrow's virtue is perfection embodied.

Two things comprise God's entire creation: the finite and the Infinite. When I, the finite, go up, it is my self-realisation. When God, the Infinite, comes down, it is His Self-manifestation. When I enter into Him, the Highest, He presents me with His Unity. When He enters into me, my lowest, I offer Him the multiplicity which He Himself entrusted to me when my soul descended to earth, Him to reveal, Him to fulfil.

All religions are in essence one, inseparable. Each religion is an unfailing path leading to the eternal Truth and is a proper manifestation of that Truth. Religion does not change, but religions must undergo vicissitudes so far as the outer form, custom, habit, ritual, circumstances and environment are concerned. "United we stand, divided we fall." This oft-quoted maxim can adequately be applied in today's talk. The united strength of all religions knows the supreme secret that no individual religion is to be looked down upon. If the united strength is wanting, then no religion can stand with its head erect. Religion is one. But it expresses itself through many, through the teeming religions.

I am deeply proud to be here at the Universalist Church, for my heart voices forth the truth that the religion which is universal is the core of all religions, and the realisation of the universal religion is not the monopoly of any particular man. Any individual, irrespective of caste, creed and nationality, can have the realisation of this universal religion if he has dynamic imagination, creative inspiration and fulfilling aspiration to assimilate the spirit of all religions.

I am a Hindu. I am proud of my Hinduism. My Hinduism, *Sanatana dharma,* the eternal religion, has taught me: *Aham brahma,* "I am the Brahman, the One without a second." You are a Christian. You are proud of your Christianity. Your divine religion has taught you: "I and my Father are one." Now if I am a Hindu in the purest sense of the term, I must be a Christian to the marrow, for deep within me what I see, feel and become is the universal Truth. What is Truth? Truth is our divine Father. A child does

137

not mind that his physical father is addressed as brother by one, uncle by another, nephew by someone else and friend by a fourth person. He is equally happy with each individual approach to his father. Similarly, when the different religions approach the Truth, our Divine Father, each in its own way, we must be supremely happy. For each religion wants the Truth and the Truth alone.

HINDUISM

"Know Thyself." This is what Hinduism stands for. This is the quintessence of Hinduism.

In a world of nervous uncertainties, in a world of dark falsehood and blind unreason, religion is one of the few things that retain their dignity. It is religion that brings man's divinity to the fore. It is religion that can inspire man to grapple with the ruthless present, reaffirm his inner strength and fight for Truth and the Hour of God.

You all know that the Hindu religion is one of the oldest religions of the world. Unlike most of the world religions, the Hindu religion has no specific founder. It is primarily based on the soul-stirring utterances of the *rishis,* the seers. A seer is one who visions the Truth and communes with the Truth.

If you want to define Hinduism, you can do so with the help of a monosyllable: Love. This Love is all-embracing and ever-growing. A staunch Hindu will say, "I can live without air, but not without God." But at the same time, if a Hindu says that he does not believe in God at all, he is still a Hindu. He feels himself to be a Hindu and others do not deny it. It is the personal choice that reigns supreme. A Hindu may worship hundreds of gods or only one. To him, God may be "Personal" or He may be "Impersonal." My young friends, I will try to explain what is meant by "Personal" and "Impersonal." An aeroplane is in the airport. You can see it. It is something concrete, material and tangible. When the plane leaves the ground and can no longer be seen, you know, nevertheless, that it is somewhere in the sky. It may be going to Canada or Japan or elsewhere. But you know that it is present on some other level, operating and functioning. Similarly, the "Impersonal" God, whom we may not see in a tangible form, we feel in our awakened consciousness, guiding and moulding us invisibly.

We have spoken of Hinduism's views on God. Now let us focus our attention on what it says about God-realisation. God-realisation is nothing short of a spiritual science which puts an end to suffering, ignorance and death. But we have to realise God for His sake and not for our sake. To seek God for our own sake is to feed our ceaseless desires in vain. But to seek God for His sake is to live in His Universal Consciousness; in other words, to be one with Him absolutely and inseparably.

The paramount question is whether God is within us all the time, whether He comes into our heart for long periods as a guest, or whether He just comes and goes. With a deep sense of gratitude, let me call upon the immortal soul of Emily Dickinson, whose spiritual inspiration im-

140

pels a seeker to know what God the Infinite precisely is. She says:

"The Infinite a sudden guest
Has been assumed to be,
But how can that stupendous come
Which never went away?"

Hinduism is called the Eternal Religion. It seeks union with God in every way known to mankind. It wants an all-fulfilling union of mankind with God, nothing more and nothing less. Its essence is tolerance. Hinduism refuses to think of world religions as separate entities. Housing within itself, as it does, all the religions of the world in its own way, it can be called, without being far from truth, a unique Fellowship of Faiths.

For a genuine Hindu, love for others is an organic part of his love for God. Cheerfully and significantly his soul will announce and sing with the dauntless spirit of Walt Whitman:

"I celebrate myself, and sing myself,
And what I assume you shall assume,
For every atom belonging to me
As good belongs to you."

The most striking feature of Hinduism is the quest for firsthand experience, nay, realisation of God. If you study the *Vedas,* the *Upanishads,* the *Bhagavad-Gita* and other Indian scriptures, you may be surprised to observe that although each emphasizes a particular view or certain ideas, they all embody fundamentally the same perfect divine Knowledge, which is God.

The salient point in the Hindu religion is uniquely expressed in the teachings of the *Isha Upanishad*: "Rejoice through renunciation." You know perfectly well that the good and the pleasant need not necessarily be the same. If you want the pleasant, you may come right up to the foot of a mango tree, but the fruits will be denied you by the owner. But if you want the good, which is in essence the Truth, the situation will be entirely different. If you want the mango, not to satisfy your greed, but to make a serious study of the fruit, the owner will be highly pleased with you. He will not only offer you a mango to study, but also tell you to eat as many as you wish.

None of us wants to play the fool; hence we must aspire for the good and do away with the pleasant once and for all. Our Goal, the fount of the highest Truth and Bliss, is open only to the Truth-lover who wants to fulfil himself in the ceaselessly delightful upward and inward journey of his soul.

A devout Hindu longs for a heart which is a perfect stranger to falsehood, a heart as vast as the world. Perhaps you may say that to have a heart of that type is next to impossible, an unattainable ideal. But I cannot concur with you. For even now such noble souls walk the earth. Your unique president, Abraham Lincoln, undoubtedly had such a heart as that. To quote your great philosopher, Ralph Waldo Emerson: "His [Lincoln's] heart was as great as the world, but there was no room in it to hold the memory of a wrong."

My brothers and sisters, I find no reason why I should fail to find in you a heart as vast as the world, empty of falsehood and ignorance, and at the same time, a heart flooded with the Truth of the Beyond.

Faith and Devotion

   Faith is God's mighty power in man.
   Devotion is man's mighty power in God.
   Faith carries man into the Heart of God.
   Devotion carries God into the heart of
man.

THE HINDUISM OF TODAY

I am a dreamer. I come from the land of dreams. I am now in a dream-boat. The name of my dream-boat is Hinduism. Day in, day out, it sails. On it sails across the Sea of Eternity. It knows no journey's end. Its goal is Immortality. The Boatman is the Dreamer Supreme. If you, my brothers and sisters, would like to sail with me in this boat, do come. I welcome you all with folded hands, with unbounded love and tears of delight. The fare demands no dollars, no cents, nothing of the sort. The fare is just sympathy, the sympathy that springs from the heart's core.

To add to the joy of our enthusiasm, a voice of a courageous dreamer, quite unexpected, is now heard echoing and re-echoing in the recesses of our memories. A century and a half ago, this dreamer saw the light of day here on Long Island, New York. He is Walt Whitman. This seer-poet, with his message of the universal "I," joins us in our momentous journey.

Our first stop is a visit to Dr. Radhakrishnan, one of the greatest living philosophers. He speaks on Hinduism:

"The Hindu attitude to religion is interesting. While fixed intellectual beliefs mark off one religion from another, Hinduism sets itself no such limits. Intellect is subordinated to intuition, dogma to experience, outer expression to inward realisation."

Keeping this in mind, let us move on to examine Hinduism. It is no doubt a great religion. But it is also a simple religion. It does not want to confuse a man or test his intellectual capacities. It does not crave his attention or solicit his favour. Significantly, what it wants from him is his soul's understanding. Hinduism wants not only to preserve but also to propagate the inner harmony of every human soul, if such is the Will of God. What it wants is to possess and be possessed by all that is best in the cultural, religious and spiritual wisdom of the world.

Although it has had its periods of inertia, Hinduism is not a static religion. A static religion would lead only to sterility and finally to death. Hinduism has, in its long history, become an emblem of flexibility, independence, creative thinking, and spontaneous innovation in both thought and action. Hinduism knows how to absorb; it knows, too, how to reject in order to sit at the feet of Truth. Hinduism is a ceaseless mounting cry for Truth. It aspires to be the essence of an all-embracing spiritual panacea to feed humanity.

India's past is remarkably rich and varied. The

same can be said of her dauntless present, which can and must provide a starting point for the golden future. The Hinduism of today is sincerely trying to discover a unique way of life in which groups of radically different racial, historical, ethical, conceptual and spiritual backgrounds can live in perfect harmony and at the same time actively collaborate in the fulfilment of one task: the marriage of Matter and Spirit. India, in its purest essence, is neither a matter-hungry nor a world-shunning country. And the tolerance with which Hinduism has always been associated is firmly rooted in sacrifice and a full recognition of other men's rights.

India acts with neither fear nor a sense of superiority. Indeed, Hinduism has become self-critical of late. Hence its improvement is dawning fast. It is true that the Hinduism of today has countless problems. It is equally true that Mother India alone must and certainly will solve all her problems. An indomitable will is energizing *Bharat Mata* (Mother India). Progress, both material and spiritual, is being effected with lightning speed. Of supreme importance, however, is the fact that the Hinduism of today is going to model itself — not on Western or Eastern or Southern or Northern patterns — but on the Infinite's own Pattern.

Here in America, we are in a land of freedom, the freedom that nourishes dynamic thoughts and dynamic movements. There in India, we are in a land of freedom, the freedom of a fertile tolerant spirituality that nourishes all religions.

147

Here we wish to reach God by running speedily, while there we wish to reach God by climbing swiftly.

Let us go and listen to a devout Hindu. He says that his father is Silence, his mother is Power. Silence feeds his consciousness. Power utilizes his consciousness. His parents teach him to breathe in the air of spiritual oneness, to feel that oneness in all human beings: indeed, in the entire creation. His parents have taught him the secret of secrets: that through meditation alone the world can be seen and felt fully and integrally. They have made him realise that his life is part and parcel of humanity. He has no race, no nation of his own. His religion is God-vision. He knows that to realise God, he has not to kill his lower self. He has just to transform it into his Higher Self. Then, behold! The Goal beckons him. Indeed, this is a new approach to and a new fulfilment of Truth. Finally, he wants not only to see God but also to be God Himself.

So our boat is sailing, dancing in tune with God's eternal, mystic cadence. We are dreamers. We are also realists and idealists. Our boat, with its heart's love, pines to touch the far-off shores of the Golden Beyond. Our boat, with its soul's peace, aspires to commune with the Breath of the Supreme.

THE QUINTESSENCE OF HINDUISM

I offer my deep sense of gratitude to our most revered Rabbi Ronald Millstein for extending to me his cordial invitation to speak on Hinduism. It is indeed a great privilege and pleasure to address this distinguished audience. I am extremely glad to learn from the Rabbi that this is a liberal synagogue. To me, the word "liberal" has a special significance. It signifies a truth as luminous and powerful as the sun, as vast as the universe. It is in our liberal understanding of all religious faiths that we can hope to achieve tolerance. Tolerance helps us to a large degree to put an end to the age-old prejudices born of ignorance.

And now my heart desires to share with you a few significant thoughts on Hinduism. Let me first tell you a short story.

A great sage of ancient India, named Bhrigu, wanted to test the three principal gods, the great Trinity of Hinduism: Brahma, Vishnu and Siva. He wished to determine who was the greatest. He approached Brahma, but showed him no respect. Brahma was very displeased with him. With the same disrespect, Bhrigu went to Siva, who became violently angry. When he went to Vishnu, he found the deity asleep. So Bhrigu put his foot on Vishnu's chest to wake him up. The god was greatly alarmed at being awakened in so rude a manner, and immediately he began to massage Bhrigu's foot affectionately, saying, "Is your foot hurt? I am so sorry." Thus Bhrigu discovered that Vishnu was the greatest of the three gods.

The tolerance shown by the god in this story was not weakness but the heart's generosity. Further, it came from a feeling of oneness. When, in our sleep, our elbow strikes some other part of our body, we do not become angry with the elbow, but massage it. Similarly, Hinduism strives to regard humanity as one great body.

Hinduism is a river that flows dynamically and untiringly. Hinduism is a tree that grows consciously and divinely. Hinduism is variety. Unique is Hinduism in her Mother aspect. She is blessed with children who cherish various conceptions of God. One of her children says: "Mother, there is no Personal God." "I see, my child," she answers. The second child says: "Mother, if there is a God, then He can only be Personal." "I see, my child," she replies. The third child says: "Mother, God is both Personal and Impersonal." "That is so, my child," she says. And now she says to them: "Be happy, my children, be happy. Stick to your own beliefs and learn through them. Grow through them and always be faithful to your ideals." Indeed, this is the Mother-Heart of Hinduism.

Hinduism clings to the inner law of life which is the common heritage of mankind. So long as one is a Truth-seeker, it does not matter if one is a theist, an atheist or an agnostic. Each human soul has its own place in the Hindu ideal of spirituality. Significant are Gandhi's words: "Hinduism is a relentless pursuit after Truth. It is the religion of Truth. Truth is God. Denial of God we have known. Denial of Truth we have not known."

HINDUISM'S PAST

It is absurd to hold that the India of the hoary past played exclusively the role of world-renunciation. Our ancients accepted life in full faith. They clearly believed in life itself as a great power.

Our Vedic parents expressed their will to live a long, radiant life when they sang:

Tach chaks ur debahitam . . .

"May we, for a hundred autumns, see
    that lustrous Eye,
God-ordained, arise before us.
May we live a hundred autumns;
May we hear for a hundred autumns;
May we speak well for a hundred au-
    tumns;
May we hold our heads high for a
    hundred autumns;
Yea, even beyond a hundred autumns."

151

In full earnest, they tried to fathom and understand the mystery of life. They accepted the earth with its joys and sorrows, its hopes and frustrations. Moreover, they wanted to live as the master and lord of life. They were therefore dauntless and uncompromising in their opposition to evil. They wanted their souls to be possessed absolutely by the Supreme and, at the same time, they aspired to serve Him in the world.

Our Vedic forebears discovered the existence of two lives: the ordinary life and the higher life. They gave due importance to physical, vital and mental activities, but with a view to entering into a higher, spiritual life, a life of more illumined knowledge, light and truth. Once established in that higher life, they knew the soul would receive absolute support from the members of its family, the body, vital, mind and heart, for its full manifestation and expression. Thus became inevitable the ideal of a special knowledge leading to the liberation of the aspiring human soul. Our ancestors were realists who felt that the spontaneous joy of life would feed the body and strengthen the soul. They knew that the secret of growth was freedom. They cried out:

Uru nastanve tan . . .

"Give freedom for our bodies,
    Give freedom for our dwelling,
    Give freedom for our life."

This was a freedom to help untie the knot of ignorance. They were positive in their acceptance of life; positive, too, in their aspiration for Immortality.

HINDUISM'S PRESENT

It is easy to insist that the India of the past was sublime while the India of today is anything but that. But they are mistaken who think that ancient Hinduism is the only part of Indian life worth study. India's present, too, has much to contribute to the world at large. Her soul's light, paying no heed to outer recognition, is playing an important role in awakening the heart of the world, and it is ultimately destined to inspire humanity with the message of truth, forgiveness and universal kindness.

Hinduism is a dynamic aspiration, divinely surcharged. In the course of its eternal journey, self-giving has been its very breath of life.

Hinduism is complex but it has always kept and forever will keep a distinct note: the note of spirituality. A true Hindu will keep his ideals burning, no matter how shattering the ephemeral changes are, no matter how powerful the destructive forces. Dr. Radhakrishnan, the philosopher-king, throws abundant light on the subject:

"When an old binding culture is being broken, when ethical standards are dissolving, when we are being aroused

out of apathy or awakened out of un-
consciousness, when there is in the air
general ferment, inward stirring, cultural crisis, then a high tide of spiritual agitation sweeps over peoples and
we sense in the horizon something
novel, something unprecedented, the
beginning of a spiritual renaissance."

The present-day world is consciously longing
for unity. Hinduism teaches that India's unity
is her oneness of spiritual vision, her integral
fulfilment. Humanity is becoming convinced of
the truth that the material, intellectual and
spiritual lives can indeed run abreast to achieve
the final victory of God here on earth.

HINDUISM: ITS SPIRITUAL SIGNIFICANCE

The ideal of Hinduism is to see all in the Self and the Self in all. A Hindu believes that each individual is a conscious manifestation of God. The spirit of selfless service is his supreme secret. A Hindu unmistakably feels that God is manifesting and perfecting Himself through each human being. Each individual soul represents a type of divinity projected by the Supreme. Each human being has a mission to fulfil on earth, and he does it at God's choice hour.

The breath of Hinduism is spirituality. Whatever a Hindu does, he does as a means to this end. It is true, as with any other individual, that he wants to accomplish all that he can here on earth. But the important thing is that he does not and cannot do anything at the expense of his spiritual life. To him, the spiritual life is the only life that can eventually garland him with the victory of perfect Perfection.

In the spiritual life, people very often use the word "sin." Here I must say that a Hindu has nothing to do with sin. He takes into consideration only two things: ignorance and Light. With his soul's light, he wants to swim across the sea of ignorance and transform his lower self into his higher Self.

Tena tyaktena bhunjita. "Enjoy through renunciation." This is the life-giving message of the Hindu seers. What is to be renounced is the train of our desires, nothing more and nothing less. In renouncing all our earth-bound desires, we can have the taste of true divine fulfilment.

I have already told you that the breath of Hinduism is spirituality. In the spiritual life, the control of the senses plays a great part. Since such is the case, let us try to clearly understand the function of the senses. A devout Hindu feels that his senses are not meant for mortification. The senses are his instruments. Their assistance is indispensable. The senses should and must function in full vigour, for the divine purpose of an all-fulfilling, integral wholeness. Then alone can true divinity dawn in human life. Self-indulgence ends in utter frustration. Poor mankind! It is so lavish in using and exhausting the pleasures of the body. Certainly man is not so lavish in his life with anything else as he is with his self-indulgence. Alas, to his utter surprise, before he exhausts the pleasures of the body, his very life exhausts itself into futile nothingness. It is high time for the brute in man to give place to the divine in him. Brutality does not conquer. It kills.

Spirituality is the all-embracing love. This love conquers man and makes him conscious of his true, inner divinity, so that he can fulfil himself and become a perfect channel for God's manifestation. This love, or this bond of love, man can create within himself in order to bind or unite himself with other individuals, other nationals, other internationals. This is what a devout Hindu feels.

No movement, no progress. Movement needs guidance. Guidance is knowledge. But man has to know that mental knowledge can only help him to a certain extent. With its help, he can go nowhere near the Goal. It is the knowledge of the soul that grants man his God-realisation.

Robert Browning said:

> "So free we seem,
> So fettered fast we are."

Man is bound *to* the finite, but he cannot be bound *by* the finite. Man has surrendered himself to time and space. But neither time nor space has compelled him to surrender. Man tries to possess the beauty of the finite. He thinks that if he can bind himself to the finite, he will be able to possess its beauty. Alas, instead of possessing, he has been possessed. Time and space have lured him. He thought he would be able to possess them with his surrender. They gladly accepted his surrender. But he has been possessed by them mercilessly. Possession is not oneness; conquest is not unity.

The vision of Hinduism is unity in diversity. First, Hinduism lovingly embraces all alien elements; second, it tries to assimilate them; third, it tries to expand itself as a whole, with a view to serving humanity and nature. Indeed, this is the sign of its life's meaningful, dynamic aspiration.

HINDUISM: THE JOURNEY OF INDIA'S SOUL

Hinduism is an inner experience; it is the experience of the soul. Hinduism is not a religion. It is the name of a culture: a self-disciplined, spiritual culture. The word "religion," in fact, is not to be found in the dictionary of a Hindu. His dictionary houses the word *dharma. Dharma,* no doubt, includes religion, but its long arms stretch far beyond the usual conception of religion. *Dharma* means the inner code of life, the deeper significance of human existence. *Dharma* is a Sanskrit word which derives from the root *dhri,* to hold. What holds man is his inner law. This inner law is a divine, all-fulfilling experience that frees man from the fetters of ignorance even while he is in the physical world.

Religion, on the other hand, is derived from the Latin verb *ligare,* to bind. The ancient Romans saw religion as a force which binds and controls man. But the ancient Indian seers felt that religion, nay, *dharma*, must release man from that which binds him, that is, his own ignorance. Man's awakened consciousness must do away with ignorance, or to be precise, must transform ignorance into the knowledge of Truth.

Sri Aurobindo says:

> "*Dharma* is the Indian conception in
> which rights and duties lose the arti-
> ficial antagonism created by a view of
> the world which makes selfishness the
> root of action, and regain their deep
> and eternal unity. *Dharma* is the basis
> of Democracy which Asia must recog-
> nize, for in this lies the distinction
> between the soul of Asia and the soul
> of Europe. Through *Dharma* the Asi-
> atic evolution fulfils itself; this is her
> secret."

In days of yore, Hinduism was known as the
Arya Dharma. Strangely enough, even now
people are not quite sure from which part of the
globe the Aryans entered India. Some, indeed,
are of the opinion that the Aryans did not come
from outside at all. Swami Vivekananda heads
the list of these firm believers.

The origin of the word "Hindu" is very
strange. It is closely associated with the river
"Sindhu," the present Indus. But the ancient
Iranians, who desired to call the Aryans by the
name of the river on which they lived, pro-
nounced it "Hindu." The Aryans seemed to like
the name and we, who are their descendants, are
enamoured and proud of the name "Hindu."

Hinduism or the Hindu *Dharma* is founded
on the spiritual teachings of the Hindu seers.
The Hindu *shastras,* or scriptures which govern

Hindu life and conduct, are illumined and surcharged with the light and power of the hallowed teachings of these ancient seers.

Many are the Hindu *shastras*. Each has made a singular, powerful contribution to the whole. The oldest and foremost of all these are the *Vedas*. They are considered the oldest written scriptures to have appeared since the dawn of civilization. The other scriptures have the *Vedas* as their only fount. The *Vedas* have another name, *Shruti,* that which is heard. They are so called because they are based on direct revelation. The authority of the *Vedas* rests on direct, inner spiritual experience that stems from divine Reality. A Hindu feels in the inmost recesses of his heart that to doubt the inner experiences of the Vedic seers is to doubt the very existence of Truth. *Vid,* to know, is the Sanskrit root of the word *Veda. Veda* actually means the Knowledge of God. As God is infinite, even so is His Knowledge. We observe in the *Vedas,* with surprise and delight, that the Truth discoveries are infinitely more important than the Truth discoverers. Unfortunately, the order of the present day is the reverse. The *Vedas* are four in number: *Rig Veda, Sama Veda, Yajur Veda* and *Atharva Veda.* Each of the *Vedas* consists of two sections: *Samhita* and *Brahmana. Samhita* contains the hymns or *mantras,* while *Brahmana* expounds their significance and appropriate application.

All the other Hindu *shastras,* other than the *Vedas* proper, are known as *Smritis. Smriti* literally mean anything that is remembered. The *Smritis* cherish their great indebtedness to the *Vedas*. They are proud of the fact that they owe their authority to the *Vedas* and to the *Vedas* alone. They have traditionally exercised great authority in laying down social and domestic laws, plying their boat between the shores of *Vidhi,* injunctions, and *Nishedha,* prohibitions, in Hindu society.

Now let us focus our attention on the *Upanishads. Upa* means near, *ni* means down, *shad* means sit. *Upanishad* refers to pupils sitting at the feet of their teacher, learning their spiritual lessons. The *Upanishads* are the philosophical and reasoned parts of the *Vedas.* They are also called *Vedanta,* end of the *Vedas.* There are two reasons for this. One is that they actually appear towards the end of the *Vedas;* the other is that they contain the spiritual essence of the *Vedas,* which is all Light and Delight. The actual number of the *Upanishads* still remains unknown. One hundred and eight have been faithfully preserved. Of these the most significant are *Isha, Kena, Katha, Prashna, Mundakya, Aitareya, Chhandogya, Brihadaranyaka and Svetasvatara.*

God-realisation abides in meditation, never in books. This is the supreme secret of the *Upanishads.* The sages and the seers in the *Upanishads* asked their pupils to meditate, only to meditate. They did not even advise their students to depend on the *Vedas* as an aid to realising God. "Meditate, the Brahman is yours! Meditate,

Immortality is yours!" At the beginning of the journey of the human soul, the Upanishadic seers cried out, *Uttisthata jagrata* . . . "Arise, awake, stop not until the Goal is reached." At the journey's end, the same seers cried out once again, *Tat twam asi,* "That Thou art."

Now let us come to the *Sad-Darshana,* the Six Systems of Indian Philosophy. These are the various schools of thought later introduced by some of the Hindu sages. The sage Jaimini's system is called *Purva Mimansa;* others are Vyasa's *Uttar Mimansa* or *Vedanta,* Kapila's *Sankhya,* Patanjali's *Yoga,* Gotama's *Nyaya,* and Kanada's *Vaisheshika.* If one studies the *Nyaya* first, then it becomes easier to fathom the other systems of thought.

All of the Six Systems were written in *sutras* or aphorisms. The sages did this because they wanted, not to expound the philosophy, but to express in the briefest possible sentences their soul-stirring revelations and to have these engraved on the memory of the aspirant. Through the passage of time, the aphorisms have been significantly adorned and armoured with countless notes and commentaries.

It is high time for us to invite Professor Max Muller to join us in today's momentous journey:

> "If I were to look over the whole world
> to find out the country most richly
> endowed with all the wealth, power
> and beauty that nature can bestow —
> in some parts a very paradise on earth

— I should point to India. . . . If I were asked under what sky the human mind has most fully developed some of its choicest gifts, has most deeply pondered on the greatest problems of life and has found solutions to some of them which well deserve the attention even of those who have studied Plato and Kant — I should point to India. And if I were to ask myself from what literature, we here in Europe, we who have been nurtured almost exclusively on the thought of Greeks and Romans, and of one Semitic race, the Jewish, may draw the corrective which is most wanted in order to make our inner life more perfect, more comprehensive, more universal, in fact more truly human, a life not for this life only, but a transfigured and eternal life — again I should point to India."

To walk along the royal path of the Six Systems of Philosophy is difficult. That path is for the learned and the select few. The common run needs an easier path. It is here that the *Puranas* come into the picture. The *Puranas* teach us the Hindu religion with inspiring and thought-provoking stories, anecdotes and parables. The *Puranas* present Hinduism in an easy, interesting, charming and convincing manner. The major difference between the *Vedas* and the

Puranas is that the Vedic gods represent the cosmic attributes of the One, while the Puranic gods represent His human attributes.

Now the *Bhagavad-Gita* or the Song Celestial demands our immediate attention. It is the scripture *par excellence.* The *Gita* is the life-breath of Hinduism. The *Gita* not only tells us to realise God, but it also tells us how. The *Gita* introduces three principal paths toward God-realisation: *Karma Yoga,* the path of action; *Jnana Yoga,* the path of knowledge; and *Bhakti Yoga,* the path of devotion. Emotional devotion and philosophical detachment not only can but must run abreast to fulfil the Divine here on earth. This sublime teaching of the *Gita* knows no equal. Without hesitation, a devout Hindu can say that the *Gita* has been the solace of his whole life and will be the solace of his death.

Certain people are heartily sick of our rituals and rites. To them, these are nothing but cheap, confused and showy affairs. But the critics will have no choice but to revise their opinions when they come to know why we perform rituals. Needless to say, we want spirituality to govern our lives, both inner and outer. Without purity of the mind, there can be no true spirituality. And for those who want purity, the performance of rituals is often an invaluable necessity. We know that when the mind is pure, illumination dawns. The subtle truths that lie beyond the range of our senses enter into our consciousness directly through the pure mind. Participation in rituals greatly aids this process. Granted, rituals are externals. But we have to know that it is the externals that bring home the truth to individuals. Rituals eventually touch the very core of our consciousness. Rituals permeate every aspect of Hindu life.

Rites, too, have been in vogue since the days of the *Atharva Veda*. Rites, if performed with an inner urge and an aspiring heart, can help us considerably to conquer the hostile forces, avert untold misfortunes and fulfil life in its divine plenitude. Indeed, this is the divine attitude. The fear of a spiritual fall threatens us only when we use the rites, or rather the magic or lesser rites, to gain selfish and undivine ends.

A word about images and symbols. We do not worship images and symbols. We worship the spirit behind them. This spirit is God. It is so easy to feel the presence of God in and through a concrete form. Through the form, one has to go to the Formless; through the finite, to the Infinite.

We worship nature. Others smile at our folly. We laugh at their ignorance. Why do we worship nature? Because we have discovered the truth. We have discovered the truth that God manifests Himself not only through nature but also *as* nature. "A thing of beauty is a joy forever," said Keats. Beauty is soul. Soul is all joy. A Hindu seeker cannot separate the aspiration of nature from the beauty and joy of the soul. Nature's aspiration and the soul's delight together create an all-loving, all-embracing and all-fulfilling perfect Perfection.

"Look at the zenith of Hindu folly!" the critics say. "For of all things in God's creation, a Hindu has to worship animals, trees, even snakes and stones." Alas, when will these men of so-called wisdom come to learn that we do not worship the stones as stones, the snakes as snakes, the trees as trees and the animals as animals. What we do is very simple, direct and spontaneous. We worship the Supreme in all these; nothing more and nothing less. With this attitude a Hindu desires to worship each and every object of the world, from the largest to the tiniest.

Let us speak of the caste system, which has been an object of ceaseless criticism. What is caste? In the deepest sense of the term, caste is unity in variety. No variety, no sign of life. Variety is essential to the cosmic evolution. All individuals cannot have the same kind of development: physical, vital, mental or spiritual. Neither is such similarity imperative. The thing of paramount importance is that each individual be given infinite opportunity and freedom to develop along his own line of growth.

In this lofty ideal, there is only one idea: to serve and be served. Each individual has his rightful place in this ideal. The caste system is to be regarded like the functioning of one's own limbs. My feet are in no way inferior to my head; one complements the other. *Brahmin* (priest, teacher and law-maker), *Kshatriya* (king and warrior), *Vaishya* (merchant, trader and agriculturist) and *Shudra* (labourer, servant and dedicated hand) are all united by their mutual service. Caste is not a division. It embodies the secret of proper understanding. And it is in proper understanding that we fulfil ourselves fully. A Hindu feels this sober truth.

True Hinduism abjures all that divides and separates. It dreams of the Supreme Truth in absolute freedom, perfect Justice in all-embracing love and the highest individual Liberation in unconditional service to humanity.

Hinduism gives due importance to all the spiritual figures of the world. It recognizes a great harmony in their teachings. Down through the ages, the firmament of India has sent forth the message of Peace, Love and Truth. It has fostered and encouraged the synthesis of all world religions. Further, Hinduism has always affirmed that the highest end of life is not to remain in any particular religion, but to outgrow religion and realise and live in Eternal Truth.

Hinduism is the embodiment of certain lofty, infallible ideals. These ideals within us live and grow, grow and live. Because of this fact, Hinduism is still a living force. It lives to lead. It leads to live.

To know Hinduism is to discover India. To discover India is to feel the Breath of the soul. To feel the Breath of the soul is to become one with God.

INDIA: HER CONSCIOUSNESS AND LIGHT

What is India's inner message to the world at large? Spirituality. What is spirituality? It is the natural way of truth that successfully communes with the Beyond here on earth.

What is India's absolutely distinctive possession? Her soul. She lives in the soul, she lives from the soul and she lives for the soul.

Where can the world find the real nature of India? In the ever-wakeful domain of the Spirit.

What has made the history of India unique? A most surprising and unusual continuity in the line of her spiritual seekers and Masters.

What does Indian spirituality teach? It teaches the world to conquer the evil of the lower nature and to go beyond the good of the higher nature.

What is Mother India's desire? It is to transcend the human way once and for all, through radical self-transmutation, and to enter into the ever-dynamic way of God.

Religion, however mighty it may be, is not and cannot be the message of India. Her message is Self-realisation.

The perfect truth of India's religion lies in its

outer and inner realisation of the One that *is*, of the One that is in the process of *becoming*.

O world, as you march on towards the deepest recesses of your heart, to your amazement, you will find Mother India to be anything but God-fearing. What then is she? She is God-loving: the God-loving soul in God's all-dreaming and all-manifesting Truth.

The soul of India feels that to be satisfied with intellectual speculation is to remain satisfied with only half the food that is actually needed for health. It is Realisation that gives one a full meal. And if one seeks Realisation, meditation and concentration are of paramount importance.

Indian philosophy, in its sublimest sense, is nothing short of the practical realisation of the Truth.

There is no more than a hyphen between the Vision of the Vedic seers and the soul of India, and between India's spirituality and the final spiritual liberation of the world.

They say that India long ago lost the Milky Way of greatness. But we know that she has now a colossal hope that the overcast sky will clear at last, revealing again the myriad points of light.

What were the chief causes of India's downfall? She neglected the body-consciousness and eschewed the material life. She narrowed her outlook and sealed herself up in the outworn rituals of the past. She clung to the festering shell of her ancient culture while killing its living, growing spirit. And India's doom was sealed the day she started these practices.

India began to rise the day she turned away from these tendencies and accepted life in all its dynamic aspects.

India will rise fully the day she becomes self-reliant. She knows well that she cannot achieve her goal if she has to depend permanently on alien help. Self-help is the best help. Self-help is God's own help in disguise.

India has within her a voice that is the self-same, all-fulfilling Voice of God. That Voice she simply must hear and obey.

What is actually meant by the emancipation of the Indian woman? It means that she must no longer be alienated from education. She must have free access to the worldwide knowledge of the present day, in addition to the sacred lore of past centuries. True education helps us to live in the integral perfection which is the very backbone of our existence on earth. The Indian woman must be given a full opportunity to develop and manifest this perfection.

The emancipation of the Indian woman also means that she must not be suppressed and dominated by man. She must be free to be herself, independent in her own right, strong and confident, a true partner and companion of man and not his drudge and serf. She must become again what she was in Vedic India, a respected and equal citizen, a glorious complement to man.

Today's India is poverty-stricken. But tomorrow's India will be prosperous. She will be a mighty wave of hope and faith. Her very thought will be stirred with a new vision. Infinite will be the possibilities on her horizon. Her sacrifice will build a more durable foundation for mankind. She will contain within herself nationalism and internationalism, becoming the true symbol of spirituality in action.

India with her spiritual power will wield a tremendous influence on future generations. This is no imagination, but vision in operation.

India and India alone is the nerve centre of the aspiring world.

India's strength is not in her arms, but in her heart. More so, it is in her seer-vision.

India tells the world that the realisation of unity is the only strength which can conquer the world.

India is the seeker of the Absolute. The *summum bonum* of life is the ideal of God-realisation. In her heart there is a burning love of God; in her mind, the service of unawakened humanity.

Consumed with desires and temptations, Europe rushed toward India to acquire her fabulous wealth. That is true. But it is equally and absolutely true that Europe's soul came to India with a spiritual seeking and an occult urge to discover what India was actually like.

India has three world-conquering weapons: Non-violence, Peace and the Wisdom which tells that she is in All as All is in her.

India's choice is character. But she must feel

that she needs personality as well.

Mother India's fear is not of atomic bombs but of her children's self-forgetful amnesia.

Unbelievably, India has perfectly reconciled in herself the two worst antagonists: renunciation and epicurianism.

Perfection was the choice of the Greeks. Proportion was the choice of the Romans. Universality is the choice of the Indians.

India is the voice that never falters. Hers is the truth that cannot be silenced by the threatening darkness of centuries. Hers is the heart that sings perpetually of the unity of mankind.

India is the vault of an ancient eternal wisdom that has a universal appeal. She is also the universal reserve bank of an ever-growing wisdom, and she is destined to be the hub and dynamo of world transformation.

Insecurity

When insecurity enters into the mind, joy departs from the heart.

EAST AND WEST

The East says: "I have seen God's Face. Now I must see His Feet." The West says: "I have seen God's Feet. Now I must see His Face."

The East says: "I have seen God's Transcendence." The West says: "I have seen God's Immanence."

The East considers life to be a continuous growth from matter to spirit. The West considers life to be a continuous growth from the simple material life to a complex and ever-expanding scientific development.

The indifferent East felt that it had nothing to hear from the West. The proud West thought that it had nothing to learn from the East.

According to the East, the West is anything but divine. According to the West, the East is idle.

It is no exaggeration to say that the East is terribly afraid of a dynamic life. Similarly, the West is terribly afraid of lone self-poise.

The East is perhaps wanting in care, detail and exactitude. But the West is wanting in breadth, vastness and universality. The East is wanting in an earthly, practical intelligence. The West is wanting in the matchless realisation of the Self.

The East feels that the mastery of one's own inner movements is the true fulfilment of life. The West feels that the mastery of the world is the true fulfilment of life.

Humility and devotion are the birthright of the East. Honesty and frankness are the birthright of the West. The combination of these four powers should be the ideal of a human being.

The East wanted to conquer the world in the name of Liberation. The West wanted to conquer the world in the name of commerce and religion.

The East has control of Spirit. The West has control of Matter. Spirit is creative, conscious existence. What is Matter? It is anything but lifeless mechanical substance. Matter is vibrant Energy which deliberately hides within itself Life and Consciousness.

The individual of the East is content to abide by the maxim, "Let me live unseen and unknown, and unlamented let me die." And, it might be added, "Let it all be done without too much exertion." The individual of the West, on the other hand, seems to desire the full expression of his individuality. He wishes to make for himself a strong and powerful position in his own world.

The East's age-long experience with the spiritual life has taught it an inner poise and equanimity in work. It can stand aside from frustration, excitement, irritation over minor upsets and all that disturbs the inner balance. It can make tranquil readjustments and proceed in the same calm tenor. This the West has yet to learn.

The West's intensive experience with material progress has taught it to be objective in work. It has learned to stand aside from favouritism, nepotism and other personal considerations in carrying out a necessary job. It can do the work for its own sake, quickly and efficiently, and with the best man-power available. This the East has yet to learn.

Indian philosophy is, in its origin, the search for the highest Truth. Only the Reality beyond the senses has been able to quench the inner thirst of the East.

European philosophy is, in its origin, an examination of ideas by the critical intellect. Until now, reason and intellect have been enough to feed the hungry West.

It is now that East and West have come to realise the need of a marriage between Mind and Spirit.

East and West may be taken as the two eyes of the same human body. The other human divisions and distinctions — racial, cultural and linguistic — are destined to disappear from the human consciousness when it is flooded with the supramental Light and Force. This is the inevitable consequence of the Hour of God that is dawning all over the world. Diversities will be there, enriched and enhanced in fullest measure. But these diversities will not be disturbances to the general consciousness. On the contrary, they will be happy and harmonious complements to a unique whole. Humanity will be a true human family in every sense of the term and in a yet unknown sense. The response to the new Light will certainly exceed human expectations.

The awakened consciousness of man is visibly tending towards the Divine. This is a most hopeful streak of light amidst the surrounding obscurities of today. This is a moment, not merely of joining hands, but of joining minds, hearts and souls. Across all physical and mental barriers between East and West, high above national standards, above even individual standards, will fly the supreme banner of Divine Oneness.

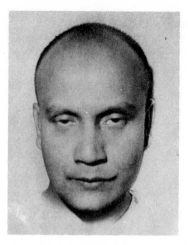

Sri Chinmoy was born in Bengal, India in 1931. While still a child he had many deep mystical experiences and at the age of twelve entered an ashram or spiritual community. Here he spent the next twenty years in intense prayer and meditation, perfecting his inner vision and reaching that rare state of oneness with God that various traditions call Enlightenment or God-realisation.

Sri Chinmoy would have been content to spend the rest of his life in a samadhi trance, maintaining only the thinnest connection with the physical world. But an inner command that he leave India and offer his realisations to aspiring humanity brought him to the United States in 1964. Since then, Sri Chinmoy spiritual Centres have been established throughout the U.S., Canada, Europe, South America, Australia and the Far East.

Besides meditating for several hours a day and guiding his various Centres, Sri Chinmoy conducts meditations twice a week for United Nations delegates and staff in New York. He delivers the monthly Dag Hammarskjold Lecture at the U.N. and is frequently invited to speak at major universities the world over. A prolific writer, Sri Chinmoy has published over 280 books of spiritual poetry, aphorisms, essays, short stories and lectures. He is also a prolific artist, having completed more than 100,000 paintings which have been exhibited at various museums, galleries and business establishments.

For information on other books by Sri Chinmoy, please contact:

Sri Chinmoy
P. O. Box 32433
Jamaica, N.Y. 11431

For additional books by Sri Chinmoy
please write to:

Sri Chinmoy
P. O. Box 32433
Jamaica, N.Y. 11431

Astrology, the Supernatural and the Beyond. A well-known Yogi and spiritual Master answers questions on astrology, the occult, psychic power, the supernatural and other cosmic forces influencing man.

paperback, $2.00

Beyond Within. A 500-page anthology of essays, discourses, stories, poems and aphorisms collected from Sri Chinmoy's writings during his ten years in the West. In this book, an illumined Yogi discusses topics such as the human psyche, meditation, will, consciousness and the higher worlds of Bliss and Light.

paperback, $6.95

Colour Kingdom. A spiritual Master of the highest order uses his own occult vision to reveal the occult meaning and significance of the different colours and shades of colour. It can be used as a practical guide for meditation and concentration exercises. Includes 51 coloured illustrations.

paperback, $5.00

Death and Reincarnation: Eternity's Voyage. A spiritual Master who has journeyed during meditation to the different planes of reality answers questions on death, reincarnation and life after death.

paperback, $2.00

Kundalini: The Mother-Power. A series of lectures on Kundalini Yoga and the awakening of hidden occult forces within man through meditation, concentration and other spiritual practices.

paperback, $2.00

Sri Chinmoy Primer. A general introduction to the spiritual life, dealing with the kinds of questions that new disciples and seekers most frequently ask a spiritual Master. Here Sri Chinmoy answers questions on meditation, mantras, diet, breathing, sex, how to choose a Guru and spiritual initiation.

paperback, $1.00

Yoga and the Spiritual Life. A comprehensive practical explanation of Yoga philosophy. Covers all aspects of the spiritual life with questions and answers on meditation and the soul.

paperback, $2.50

INDEX

INDEX

Absolute, 22, 96, 172

acceptance, 53, 55; of humanity, 16; of the spiritual life, 49; of our earthly existence and Karma Yoga, 59; of life, 71, 151, 171; and Perfection, 76; of the earth, 152

achievement, 92, 98; of peace, 14; of immortality, 35; of Perfection, 76; of God's all-pervading Consciousness, 105; and manifestation, 97-98

action, and inaction, Gita's view and meaning of, 10; correct attitude towards, 10; made more real and effective, 10; successful action, 10; to please the Inner Pilot (God, the soul), 10, 23; and Peace, 13; and the sea of Peace, 14; divine and undivine, 16; is secret and sacred and meant for our own progress, 23; and responsibility, 27; and parts of the

body, 32-33; and purity, 39; and Agami Karma, 44; and outer, inner life, 47; necessity of, 51; and God, 51; and Karma Yoga, 59, 60; and Karma Yogi, 61; from the intuitive mind, 93; and Creation, 136

Adam and Eve, 27

Agami Karma, *defined*, 44

Aham Brahma, *meaning of*, 137

aim of life, chapter on, 47-50; stated, 47, 48, 49, 52; according to Sri Ramakrishna, 52; Hinduism's view of, 168

America, darkness and Light battle, 67, 68; land of freedom and India, 147-148

analogies, flute and flutist and our attitude towards God, 2; master-servant and soul-mind, 9-10; individual-collective meditation and instrument-symphonic unity, 26; human child and the di-

meditation, 27; and the Bhakta, 57-58, 58; and the Karma Yogin, 60; a path to God, 85, 165; and repeating the word God, 95; the birth-right of the East, 176

Dharma, *meaning of,* 159; Sri Aurobindo on, 160

difficulties, in meditation, 28

discrimination, 15

disease, 27, 75

disharmony, 130

divine, the Divine, 21, 39, 44, 51, 53, 105, 118, 124, 178, Mother aspect of, 18, love for, 22, fulfilment of, 55, 119, 121, 127, 165, quality of, 75; individuality, 21; hero, 28-29, 60; lubricant, 37; Joy, 40; Play, 44, 82; Door of the, 51; representative, 55-56; will, 116, 119; mission, 117

divinity, 16, 52, 53, 125-126; 139, 156

doubt, 18, 57, 82, 161, *defined,* 31; basis of, 31

dream, 86, 115, 145

earth, 1, 55, 64, 68, 93, 120, 125; consciousness, 68

East, essence of and comparison with the West, 175-178

education, true, 171

effort, conscious and unconscious, 28; necessity of, 69-70

ego, man identifies himself with, 8; steps to deal with, 9; and our return to the Blissful, 18; *defined* and described, 104; how it was born, how it came into existence, what it tries to do, 104-105; how we may weaken and ultimately subdue, 105; demands of, 118-119

eight strides of Yoga, 19

elite, role of, 69

"enjoy through renunciation," message of Hindu seers, 156

enlightened souls, 69

epicurianism, 173

equanimity, 176-177

escape, 62, 75

esoteric, reality, 47; traditions, 102

eternal, 13, 36, 125; journey, 25; now, 49; Truth, 168

eternity, 6, 13, 25, 59, 124, 132

Europe, in quote by Max Muller, 164; and India, 172; its philosophy, 177

evil, 75, 152, 169

evolution, soul's awareness of, 25; Darwin's theory of, 44; spiritual evolution, *meaning of,* 44-45; *defined,* 47, 136; beginning of a new and higher cycle of, 68; of the individual soul, 101, 116-117, 126; degrees of, 119-120; necessity of variety in, 167

present-day world, 21; earthly, 21; and surrender, 21; realisation's view of, 36; and God, 40; we already have, 41-42; is killed by, 130; wants, 130; *defined,* 130; in America and India, 147; the secret of growth, 152; Vedic message on, 152; role of, 153; necessity for individual development, 167

ulfilment, and marriage, 3-4; 73, 74; role of prayer in, 14; and surrender, 23, 74; and God, 28, 63, 74, 84, 101; and aspiration, 32; of soul's mission, 32, 33, 117; individual and collective, 32; source of, 33; and realisation, 36; and the liberated soul, 44; of the outer reality, 47; of the inner reality, 47; and spirituality, 51; and the Jnana Yogin, 61; and the material world, 68; destined, 68; and America, 69; and soul's path, 86; in the outer world, 92; and chanting AUM, 95; and vision, 98; and the ego, 105, 119; and soul's selection of body, 116; of the Divine, 117-118, 119, 121, 127, 165; and reincarnation, 120; of matter and Spirit, 120, 147; and the physical consciousness, 121; and the soul's

choice of experiences, 121, and Truth, 133, 148; and willpower, 135; and the goal, 142; how to obtain, 148; and India's unity, 154; and renunciation, 156; and love, 156; and teaching of the Gita, 165; and caste, 167-168

Full in the Void, 14-15

future, God's view of, 63; and plans, 63, 64, 97; and vision, 98

go deep within, 32, 40, 88, 91, 100

goal, is within us, 7, 10; how to reach, 10, 148, 157; *defined,* 18, 142; and Yogic paths, 27; and aspiration, 31; and the Jnana Yogin, 61; and spiritual experiences, 83; impediments to reaching, 124; is open to, 142; of Hinduism, 145; and transformation, 148; and mental knowledge, 157

God, mentioned, 3, 7, 8, 17, 18, 19, 22, 33, 40, 44, 51, 57, 58, 59, 64, 65, 97, 100, 108, 129, 148, 166; *defined,* 7, 18, 22, by Emerson, 44. 57, 64, 65, 76, 100, by Gandhi, 151. 166; as Friend, Guide, Master, 1; as Father, 2, 61, 101; as Master, Spirit, 2; God-real-

hunger, for spiritual food, 8

"I," the real I and the body, 36
"I and my Father are one," statement of Christ compared with the Hindu tradition, 101, 137
"I can see God," and the third eye, 109
ideal, of the heart, 142; and the Mother's message, 150; of special knowledge, 152; and the true Hindu, 153; of Hinduism, 155; for growth, 167; and Hinduism, 168; of God-Realisation, 172; of a human being, 176
ignorance, and the ego, 8, 104; its destruction, 15; freedom from, 15, 26, 35, 36, 40, 48, 112, 155-156, 159; and realisation, 26, 35; and collective meditation, 28; and Vedic realisation, 35, 152-153; and God, 40; and renunciation, 48; and the Jnana Yogin, 62; and the earth-consciousness, 68; and the caste-system, 73; and the soul, 112, 116, 121; and the heart, 143; source of prejudice, 149; and sin, 155; and dharma, 159; and worship of nature, 166
illumination, *defined,* 27; source of, 36, 81, 165; necessity

of, 130; illumined and divine nature, 26
illusion, see Maya
images, and worship, 166
imagination, and exercise for purity, 41; necessity of, 48; and realisation, 137
immorality, 134
immortal, 36, 44; immortality, 7, 62, aphorism on, 6, and realisation, 37, and the Lord, 52, source of, 52, 120, 152-153, 162-163, God's song of, 59, and the supreme sacrifice, 74, and matter spiritualised, 120, and religion, 134, goal of Hinduism, 145, and our Vedic forebears, 153, and meditation, 162-163
impairment, to our evolving spiritual consciousness, 69
imperfection, and fault-finding, 15-16; positive approach to, 41; view of the world, 64; man's interpretation, basis of, 64-65; and the path of escape, 75; victory over, 75; soul's acceptance of, 116; soul's sympathy for, 118; in definition of sin, 136
incarnation, 84, 123-124
independence, and the Mother, 18
India, 22, 69, 70, 71, 96, 147, 149, 151, 153, 168, 169-

189

group meditation, 28; from hope and courage, 32; necessity of, 48, 51; and the Jnana Yogin, 61; to action, 63· and book study, 80-81; and choosing a path, 85-86; from repetition of AUM, 94; from a particular mantra, 96; from the soul, 118; religious, *defined,* 131, and perfection of philosophy, 134-135; and realisation, 137; from religion, 139; from Emily Dickinson, 140-141; and India, 153

instruction, necessity for Jnana Yogin, 61; of the soul, 116

instrument, flute and Flutist, analogies to attitude towards God, 2; in aphorism, 15; meditation analogy using, 26; and spontaneous faith, 80; and operating from a particular plane of consciousness, 93; of the omnipotent power, 131; and the senses, 156

intellect, view of, Katha Upanishad's, 122; use of, Hinduism's, according to Dr. Radhakrishnan, 146; intellectual speculation, view of, India's soul, 170; and European philosophy, 177

intuition, source of knowledge and Sri Chinmoy, 91; and movement toward success,

97; and oneness with God, 97; *defined* and described, 99, 129; and religion, 129-130; in quote from Dr. Radhakrishnan, 146

Isha Upanishad, message from, 142

Japa, *meaning of,* 40; value of, 40

Jnana Yoga, a path to God, 27, 56; of three main gates, 56; *defined*, described and compared with other Yogic paths, 61-62; and the Gita, 165

journey, 114; aspects of, 3, 19; and achieving peace, 14; spiritual help along, 23; eternal, of the soul, 25; end of, and aspiration, 31; inevitability of mistakes along, 49; and renunciation, 83; how to begin, 86; beginning of, and soul's selection of body, 115; obstacles along, 124; is there any end? 145; visit by Walt Whitman and Dr. Radhakrishnan, 145-146; and Hinduism, 153; message from seers, 163; visit by Professor Max Muller, 163-164

joy, 145; source of, 16; and our return home, 18; and collective meditation, 28; and desire, 35; and realisa-

mysteries, incapacity of science in solving, 52-53; can be known by spiritual men, 53; a way to discover, 87; and the Vedic seers, 152

Nama-Rupa, its *meaning* and explanation, 99-100
natural, state of consciousness, 31, and spontaneous, life, 52
nature, divine and undivine, effect of, 26; and science, 134; worship of God in, discussed, 166; higher and lower, India's teaching about, 169
nature's dance, ending in Samadhi, 19
Nectar, 8; *defined,* 11
need, of purity, 39
Neti, Neti, *meaning of,* explanation, 62
New York, the soul of, 120
Niyama, *defined,* 19
non-attachment, and peace, 48
non-violence, of India, 172

objectivity, Western attitude, 177
obstacles, to reaching the Goal, 124
ocean, in analogy to individual and Universal Soul, 17; analogy to individual and the whole, 26; a Bhakta's attitude to God, 58; in medi-

tation, explanation and proper understanding of, 90
omnipotent power, in surrender, 21; and problems, 131
oneness, sign of spiritual fitness, 17; ultimate stage in yoga, 19; goal of meditation, 26; and realisation, 35; and true spirituality, 53; and surrender, 74; with God's Will, 84; and Law of Karma, 85; basis for intuition, 97; and vision and fulfilment, 98; in religion, 130; and Hinduism, 148, 168; backbone of tolerance, 150; of India's unity, 154; contrasted with possession, 157; the future of East and West, 178
one-pointed, meditation, result of, 27
outer, life, and the mind, 9, qualities of, in comparison with inner life, 47, how to simplify, 51-52; world, 47, and God, 9, and discrimination, 15, synthesis with the inner world, how to create, 91-92; being, synthesis with the inner being, how to create, 91; and operating from a particular plane of consciousness, 93, and chanting AUM, 94

200

revelation, and meaning of realisation, 35; and inner joy, 40; and the Eternal Now, 49-50

rites, *meaning,* 165-166; use of, 165-166

rituals, *meaning,* 165-166; use of, 165-166

Romans, and India, their choices, 173

sacrifice, of wife and husband, 3-4; of Divine Love, 78; basis of aspiration, 91; tolerance of India, 147; India of the future, 172

Sad-Darshana, discussed, 163

sage, Kapila, and theory of spiritual evolution, 125; Bhrigu, 149-150; Jaimini, 163; and others, 163

salvation, 27

samadhi, *defined,* 19

Sanatana dharma, "Eternal Religion," Hinduism, 137

Sanchita Karma, *defined,* 43

Sanskrit, words, AUM, 94, special significance of, 94, origin of word karma, 126

"Sarvam Khalvidam Brahma," *meaning,* 36

Sat-Chit-Ananda, *meaning of* and explanation, 103

Saviour, 27

sceptics, 5

science, its vision limited, 52; incapable of solving inner

mysteries, 53; and yoga, 55; and realisation, 140; effect upon our ideas, 102; and Kingdom of Heaven, 102; in locating heart, 121-122; and religion, 134; and Western view of life, 175

scriptures, not needed to realise God, 49; compared to direct knowledge, 82; Indian, 141-142; teachings of ancient seers, 160; oldest is Vedas, 161; other than Vedas, Smriti, 161-163; see also Hindu shastras

sea of, silence, while acting, 10; peace, amidst daily activities, 14; liberation, 47; ignorance, and Jnana Yogin, 62; knowledge and light, 62; ignorance, and Hinduism, 155-156

secret, "That Thou Art," 26; of karma, 43; of chanting AUM, 95; of secrets, in Hindu life, 148; of growth, 152

seeing, self-illumining Light, 7; and inmost heart, 8; and being Godlike, 81

seeker, 28, 35; beginner, 3; attaining realisation, 37; having a personal teacher, 87; and the Hindu ideal, 151; a Hindu, and mature aspiration, 166; and India's history, 169; India, a seeker, 172